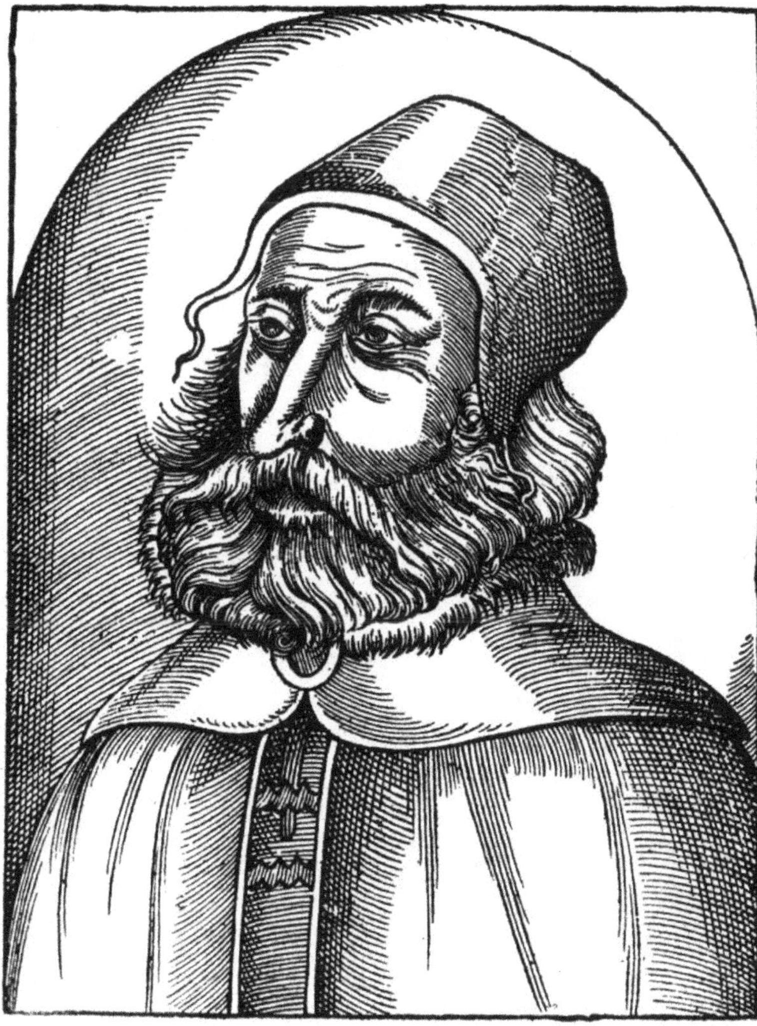

BOOK I

1 Since feeling and voluntary motion are peculiar to animals, whilst growth and nutrition are common to plants as well, we may look on the former as effects of the soul and the latter as effects of nature. And if there be anyone who allows a share in soul to plants as well, and separates the two kinds of soul, naming the kind in question vegetative, and the other sensory, this person is not saying anything else, although his language is somewhat unusual. We, however, for our part, are convinced that the chief merit of language is clearness, and we know that nothing detracts so much from this as do unfamiliar terms; accordingly we employ those terms which the bulk of people are accustomed to use, and we say that animals are governed at once by their soul and by their nature, and plants by their nature alone, and that growth and nutrition are the effects of nature, not of soul.

2 Thus we shall enquire, in the course of this treatise, from what faculties these effects themselves, as well as any other effects of nature which there may be, take their origin. First, however, we must distinguish and explain clearly the various terms which we are going to use in this treatise, and to what things we apply them; and this will prove to be not merely an explanation of terms but at the same time a demonstration of the effects of nature. When, therefore, such and such a body undergoes no change from its existing state, we say that it is at rest; but, notwithstanding, if it departs from this in any respect, we then say that in this respect it undergoes motion.

Accordingly, when it departs in various ways from its preexisting state, it will be said to undergo various kinds of motion. Thus, if that which is white becomes black, or what is black becomes white, it undergoes motion in respect to color; or if what was previously sweet now becomes bitter, or, conversely, from being bitter now becomes sweet, it will be said to undergo motion in respect to flavor; to both of these instances, as well as to those previously mentioned, we shall apply the term qualitative motion. And further, it is not only things which are altered in regard to color and flavor which, we say, undergo motion; when a warm thing becomes cold, and a cold warm, here too we speak of motion; similarly, also when anything moist becomes dry, or dry moist. Now, the common term which we apply to all these cases is alteration. This is one kind of motion. But there is another king which occurs in bodies which change their position, or as we say, pass from one place to another; the name of this is transference. These two kinds of motion, then, are simple and primary, while compounded from them we have growth and decay, as when a small thing becomes bigger, or a big thing smaller, each retaining at the same time its particular form.

And two other kinds of motion are genesis and destruction, genesis being a coming into existence, and destruction being the opposite. Now, common to all kinds of motion is change from the preexisting state, while common to all conditions of rest is retention of the preexisting state. The Sophists, however, while allowing that bread in turning into blood becomes changed as regards sight, taste, and touch, will not agree that this change occurs in reality. Thus, some of them hold that all such phenomena are tricks and illusions of our senses; the senses, they say, are affected now in one way, now in another, whereas the underlying substance does not admit of any of these changes to which the names are given. Others (such as Anaxagoras) will have it that the qualities do exist in it, but that they are unchangeable and immutable from eternity to eternity, and that these apparent alterations are brought about by separation and combination. Now, if I were to go out of my way to confute these people, my subsidiary task would be greater than my main one.

Thus, if they do not know all that has been written, *On Complete Alteration of Substance* by Aristotle, and after him by Chrysippus, I must beg them to make themselves familiar with these men's writings. If, however, they know these, and yet willingly prefer the worse views to the better, they will doubtless consider my arguments foolish also. I have shown elsewhere that these opinions were shared by Hippocrates, who lived much earlier than Aristotle. In fact, all those known to us who have been both physicians and philosophers Hippocrates was the first who took in hand to demonstrate that there are, in all, four mutually interacting qualities, and that to the operation of these is due the genesis and destruction of all things that come into and pass out of being. Nay, more; Hippocrates was also the first to recognise that all these qualities undergo an intimate mingling with one another; and at least the beginnings of the proofs to which Aristotle later set his hand are to be found first in the writings of Hippocrates. As to whether we are to suppose that the substances as well as their qualities undergo this intimate mingling, as Zeno of Citium afterwards declared, I do not think it necessary to go further into this question in the present treatise; for immediate purposes we only need to recognize the complete alteration of substance. In this way, nobody will suppose that bread represents a kind of meeting-place for bone, flesh, nerve, and all the other parts, and that each of these subsequently becomes separated in the body and goes to join its own kind; before any separation takes place, the whole of the bread obviously becomes blood; (at any rate, if a man takes no other food for a prolonged period, he will have blood enclosed in his veins all the same). And clearly this disproves the view of those who consider the elements unchangeable, as also, for that matter, does the oil which is entirely used up in the flame of the lamp, or the faggots which, in a somewhat longer time, turn into fire. I said, however, that I was not going to enter into an argument with these people, and it was only because the example was drawn from the subject-matter of medicine, and because I need it for the present treatise, that I have mentioned it.

We shall then, as I said, renounce our controversy with them, since those who wish may get a good grasp of these views of the ancients from our own personal investigations into these matters. The discussion which follows we shall devote entirely, as we originally proposed, to an enquiry into the number and character of the faculties of Nature, and what is the effect which each naturally produces. Now, of course, I mean by an effect that which has already come into existence and has been completed by the activity of these faculties—for example, blood, flesh, or nerve. And activity is the name I give to the active change or motion, and the cause of this I call a faculty. Thus, when food turns into blood, the motion of the food is passive, and that of the vein active. Similarly, when the limbs have their position altered, it is the muscle which produces, and the bones which undergo the motion. In these cases I call the motion of the vein and of the muscle an activity, and that of the food and the bones a symptom or affection, since the first group undergoes alteration and the second group is merely transported. One might, therefore, also speak of the activity as an effect of Nature—for example, digestion, absorption, blood-production; one could not, however, in every case call the effect an activity; thus flesh is an effect of Nature, but it is, of course, not an activity. It is, therefore, clear that one of these terms is used in two senses, but not the other.

3 It appears to me, then, that the vein, as well as each of the other parts, functions in such and such a way according to the manner in which the four qualities are mixed. There are, however, a considerable number of not undistinguished men—philosophers and physicians—who refer action to the Warm and the Cold, and who subordinate these, as passive, the Dry and the Moist; Aristotle, in fact, was the first who attempted to bring back the causes of the various special activities to these principles, and he was followed later by the Stoic school. These latter, of course, could logically make active principles of the Warm and the Cold, since they refer the change of the elements themselves into one another to certain diffusions and condensations. This does not hold of Aristotle, however; seeing that he employed the four qualities to explain the genesis of the elements, he ought properly to have also referred the causes of all the special activities to these. How is it that he uses the four qualities in his book *On Genesis and Destruction,* whilst in his *Meteorology,* his *Problems,* and many other works he uses the two only? Of course, if anyone were to maintain that in the case of animals and plants the Warm and the Cold are more active, the Dry and Moist less so, he might perhaps have even Hippocrates on his side; but if he were to say that this happens in all cases, he would, I imagine, lack support, not merely from Hippocrates, but even from Aristotle himself—if, at least, Aristotle chose to remember what he himself taught us in his work *On Genesis and Destruction,* not as a matter of simple statement, but with an accompanying demonstration. I have, however, also investigated these questions, in so far as they are of value to a physician, in my work *On Temperaments.*

4 The so-called blood-making faculty of the veins, then, as well as all the other faculties, fall within the category of relative concepts; primarily because the faculty is the cause of the activity, but also, accidentally, because it is the cause of the effect. But, if the cause is relative to something—for it is the cause of what results from it, and of nothing else—it is obvious that the faculty also falls into the category of the relative; and so long as we are ignorant of the true essence of the

cause which is operating, we call it a faculty. Thus, we say that there exists in the veins a blood-making faculty, as also a digestive faculty in the stomach, a pulsatile faculty in the heart, and in each of the other parts a special faculty corresponding to the function or activity of that part. If, therefore, we are to investigate methodically the number and kinds of faculties, we must begin with the effects; for each of these effects comes from a certain activity, and each of these again is preceded by a cause.

5 The effects of Nature, then, while the animal is still being formed in the womb, are all the different parts of its body; and after it has been born, an effect in which all parts share is the progress of each to its full size, and thereafter its maintenance of itself as long as possible. The activities corresponding to the three effects mentioned are necessarily three—one to each—namely, Genesis, Growth, and Nutrition. Genesis, however, is not a simple activity of Nature, but is compounded of alteration and of shaping. That is to say, in order that bone, nerve, veins, and all other [tissues] may come into existence, the underlying substance from which the animal springs must be altered; and in order that the substance so altered may acquire its appropriate shape and position, its cavities, outgrowths, attachments, and so forth, it has to undergo a shaping or formative process. One would be justified in calling this substance which undergoes alteration the material of the animal, just as wood is the material of a ship, and wax of an image. Growth is an increase and expansion in length, breadth, and thickness of the solid parts of the animal (those which have been subjected to the molding or shaping process). Nutrition is an addition to these, without expansion.

6 Let us speak then, in the first place, of Genesis, which, as we have said, results from alteration together with shaping. The seed having been cast into the womb or into the earth (for there is no difference), then, after a certain definite period, a great number of parts become constituted in the substance which is being generated; these differ as regards moisture, dryness, coldness and warmth, and in all the other qualities which naturally derive therefrom. These derivative qualities, you are acquainted with, if you have given any sort of scientific consideration to the question of genesis and destruction. For, first and foremost after the qualities mentioned come the other so-called tangible distinctions, and after them those which appeal to taste, smell, and sight. Now, tangible distinctions are hardness and softness, viscosity, friability, lightness, heaviness, density, rarity, smoothness, roughness, thickness and thinness; all of these have been duly mentioned by Aristotle. And of course you know those which appeal to taste, smell, and sight. Therefore, if you wish to know which alterative faculties are primary and elementary, they are moisture, dryness, coldness, and warmth, and if you wish to know which ones arise from the combination of these, they will be found to be in each animal of a number corresponding to its sensible elements. The name sensible elements is given to all the homogeneous parts of the body, and these are to be detected not by any system, but by personal observation of dissections. Now Nature constructs bone, cartilage, nerve, membrane, ligament, vein, and so forth, at the first stage of the animal's genesis, employing at this task a faculty which is, in general terms, generative and alterative, and, in more detail, warming, chilling, drying, or moistening; or such as spring from the blending of these, for example, the bone-producing, nerve-producing, and cartilage-producing faculties (since for the sake of clearness these names must be used as well).

Now the peculiar flesh of the liver is of this kind as well, also that of the spleen, that of the kidneys, that of the lungs, and that of the heart; so also is the proper substance of the brain, stomach, gullet, intestines, and uterus is a sensible element, of similar parts all through, simple, and uncompounded. That is to say, if you remove from each of the organs mentioned its arteries, veins, and nerves, the substance remaining in each organ is, from the point of view of the senses, simple and elementary. As regards those organs consisting of two dissimilar coats, of which each is simple, of these organs the coats are the elements—for example, the coats of the stomach, oesophagus, intestines, and arteries; each of these two coats has an alterative faculty peculiar to it, which has engendered from it the menstrual blood of the mother. Thus the special alterative faculties in each animal are of the same number as the elementary parts; and further, the activities must necessarily correspond each to one of the special parts, just as each part has its special use—for example, those ducts which extend from the kidneys into the bladder, and which are called ureters; for these are not arteries, since they do not pulsate nor do they consist of two coats; and they are not veins, since they neither contain blood, nor do their coats in any way resemble those of veins; from nerves they differ still more than from the structures mentioned. "What, then, are they?" someone asks—as though every part must necessarily be either an artery, a vein, a nerve, or a complex of these, and as though the truth were not what I am now stating, namely, that every one of the various organs has its own particular substance. For in fact the two bladders—that which receives the urine, and that which receives the yellow bile—not only differ from all other organs, but also from one another. Further, the ducts which spring out like kinds of conduits from the gall-bladder and which pass into the liver have no resemblance either to arteries, veins or nerves. But these parts have been treated at a greater length in my work *On the Anatomy of Hippocrates,* as well as elsewhere.

As for the actual substance of the coats of the stomach, intestine, and uterus, each of these has been rendered what it is by a special alterative faculty of Nature; while the bringing of these together, therewith of the structures which are inserted into them, the outgrowth into the intestine, the shape of the inner cavities, and the like, have all been determined by a faculty which we call the shaping or formative faculty; this faculty we also state to be artistic—nay, the best and highest art—doing everything for some purpose, so that there is nothing ineffective or superfluous, or capable of being better disposed. This, however, I shall demonstrate in my work *On the Use of Parts.*

7 Passing now to the faculty of Growth let us first mention that this, too, is present in the foetus in utero as is also the nutritive faculty, but that at that stage these two faculties are, as it were, handmaids to those already mentioned, and do not possess in themselves supreme authority. When, however, the animal has attained its complete size, then, during the whole period following its birth and until the acme is reached, the faculty of growth is predominant, while the alterative and nutritive faculties are accessory—in fact, act as its handmaids. What, then, is the property of this faculty of growth? To extend in every direction that which has already come into existence—that is to say, the solid parts of the body, the arteries, veins, nerves, bones, cartilages, membranes, ligaments, and the various coats which we have just called elementary, homogeneous, and simple. And I shall state in what way they gain this extension in every direction, first giving an illustration for the sake of clearness. Children take the bladders of pigs, fill them with air, and then rub them on ashes near the fire, so as to warm, but not to injure them. This is a common game in the district of Ionia, and among not a few other nations. As they rub, they sing songs, to a certain measure, time, and rhythm, and all their words are an exhortation to the bladder to increase in size. When it appears to them fairly well distended, they again blow air into it and expand it further; then they rub it again. This they do several times, until the bladder seems to them to have become large enough. Now, clearly, in these doings of the children, the more the interior cavity of the bladder increases in size, the thinner, necessarily, does its substance become. But, if the children were able to bring nourishment to this thin part, then they would make the bladder big in the same way that Nature does. As it is, however, they cannot do what Nature does, for to imitate this is beyond the power not only of children, but of any one soever; it is a property of Nature alone. It will now, therefore, be clear to you that nutrition is a necessity for growing things. For if such bodies were distended, but not at the same time nourished, they would take on a false appearance of growth, not a true growth. And further, to be distended in all directions belongs only to bodies whose growth is directed by Nature; for those which are distended by us undergo this distension in one direction but grow less in the others; it is impossible to find a body which will remain entire and not be torn through whilst we stretch it in the three dimensions. Thus, Nature alone has the power to expand a body in all directions so that it remained unruptured and preserves completely its previous form. Growth is then, and it cannot occur without the nutriment which flows to the part and is worked up into it.

8 We have, then, it seems, arrived at the subject of Nutrition, which is the third and remaining consideration which we proposed at the outset. For, when the matter which flows to each part of the body in the form of nutriment is being worked up into it, this activity is nutrition, and its cause is the nutritive faculty. Of course, the kind of activity here involved is also an alteration, but not an alteration like that occurring at the stage of genesis. For in the latter case something comes into existence which did not exist previously, while in nutrition the inflowing material becomes assimilated to that which has already come into existence. Therefore, the former kind of alteration has with reason been termed genesis, and the latter, assimilation.

9 Now, since the three faculties of Nature have been exhaustively dealt with, and the animal would appear not to need any others (being possessed of the means for growing, for attaining completion, and for maintaining itself as a long a time as possible), this treatise might seem to be already complete, and to constitute an exposition of all the faculties of Nature. If, however, one considers that it has not yet touched upon any of the parts of the animal (I mean the stomach, intestines, liver, and the like), and that it has not dealt with the faculties resident in these, it will seem as though merely a kind of introduction had been given to the practical parts of our teaching. For the whole matter is as follows: Genesis, growth, and nutrition are the first, and, so to say, the principal effects of Nature; similarly also the faculties which produce these effects—the first faculties—are three in number, and are the most dominating of all. But as has already been shown, these need the service both of each other, and of yet different faculties. Now, these which the faculties of generation and growth require have been stated. I shall now say what ones the nutritive faculty requires.

10 For I believe that I shall prove that the organs which have to do with the disposal of the nutriment, as also their faculties, exist for the sake of this nutritive faculty. For since the action of this faculty is assimilation, and it is impossible for anything to be assimilated by, and to change into anything else unless they already possess a certain community and affinity in their qualities, therefore, in the first place, any animal cannot naturally derive nourishment from any kind of food, and secondly, even in the case of those from which it can do so, it cannot do this at once. Therefore, by reason of this law, every animal needs several organs for altering the nutriment. For in order that the yellow may become red, and the red yellow, one simple process of alteration is required, but in order that white may become black, and the black white, all the intermediate stages are needed. So also, a thing which is very soft cannot all at once become very hard, nor vice versa; nor, similarly can anything which has a very bad smell suddenly become quite fragrant, nor again, can the converse happen. How, then, could blood ever turn into bone, without having first become, as far as possible, thickened and white? And how could bread turn into blood without having gradually parted with its whiteness and gradually acquired redness? Thus it is quite easy for blood to become flesh; for, if Nature thicken it to such an extent that it acquires a certain consistency and ceases to be fluid, it thus becomes original newly-formed flesh; but in order that blood may turn into bone, much time is needed and much elaboration and transformation of the blood. Further, it is quite clear that bread, and, more particularly lettuce, beet, and the like, require a great deal of alteration, in order to become blood. This, then, is one reason why there are so many organs concerned in the alteration of food.

A second reason is the nature of the superfluities. For, as we are unable to draw any nourishment from grass, although this is possible for cattle, similarly we can derive nourishment from radishes, albeit not to the same extent as form meat; for almost the whole of the latter is mastered by our natures; it is transformed and altered and constituted useful blood; but, notwithstanding, in the radish, what is appropriate and capable of being altered (and that only with difficulty, and with much labour) is the very smallest part; almost the whole of it is surplus matter, and passes through the digestive organs, only a very little being taken up into the veins as blood—nor is this itself entirely utilisable blood. Nature, therefore, had need of a second process of separation for the superfluities in the veins. Moreover, these superfluities need, on the one hand, certain fresh routes to conduct them to the outlets, so that they may not spoil the useful substances, and they also need certain reservoirs, as it were, in which they are collected till they reach a sufficient quantity, and are then discharged. Thus, then, you have discovered bodily parts of a second kind, consecrated in this case to the [removal of the] superfluities of the food. There is, however, also a third kind, for carrying the pabulum in every direction; these are like a number of roads intersecting the whole body. Thus there is one entrance—that through the mouth—for all the various articles of food. What receives nourishment, however, is not one single part, but a great many parts, and these widely separated; do not be surprised, therefore, at the abundance of organs which Nature has created for the purpose of nutrition. For those of them which have to do with alteration prepare the nutriment suitable for each part; others separate out the superfluities; some pass these along, others store them up, others excrete them; some, again, are paths for the transit in all directions of the utilisable juices. So, if you wish to gain a thorough acquaintance with all the faculties of Nature, you will have to consider each one of these organs. Now in giving an account of these we must begin with those effects of Nature, together with their corresponding parts and faculties, which are closely connected with the purpose to be achieved.

11 Let us once more, then, recall the actual purpose for which Nature has constructed all these parts. Its name, as previously stated, is nutrition, and the definition corresponding to the name is: an assimilation of that which nourishes to that which receives nourishment. And in order that this may come about, we must assume a preliminary process of adhesion, and for that, again, one of presentation. For whenever the juice which is destined to nourish any of the parts of the animal is emitted from the vessels, it is in the first place dispersed all through this part, next it is presented, and next it adheres, and becomes completely assimilated. The so-called white [leprosy] shows the difference between assimilation and adhesion, in the same way that the kind of dropsy which some people call anasarca clearly distinguishes presentation from adhesion. For, of course, the genesis of such a dropsy does not come about as do some of the conditions of atrophy and wasting, from an insufficient supply of moisture; the flesh is obviously moist enough,—in fact it is thoroughly saturated,—and each of the solid parts of the body is in a similar condition. While, however, the nutriment conveyed to the part does undergo presentation, it is still too watery, and is not properly transformed into a juice, nor has it acquired that viscous and agglutinative quality which results from the operation of innate heat; therefore, adhesion cannot come about, since, owing to this abundance of thin, crude liquid, the pabulum runs off and easily slips away from the solid parts of the body. In white [leprosy], again, there is adhesion of the nutriment but no real assimilation. From this it is clear that what I have just said is correct, namely, that in that part which is to be nourished there must first occur presentation, next adhesion, and finally assimilation proper. Strictly speaking, then, nutriment is that which is actually nourishing, while the quasi-nutriment which is not yet nourishing (e.g. matter which is undergoing adhesion or presentation) is not, strictly speaking, nutriment, but is so called only by an equivocation. Also, that which is still contained in the veins, and still more, that which is in the stomach, from the fact that it is destined to nourish if properly elaborated, has been called "nutriment." Similarly we call the various kinds of food "nutriment," not because they are already nourishing the animal, nor because they exist in the same state as the material which actually is nourishing it, but because they are able and destined to nourish it if they be properly elaborated. This was also what Hippocrates said, viz., *Nutriment is what is engaged in nourishing, as also is quasi-nutriment, and what is destined to be nutriment.* For to that which is already being assimilated he gave the name of nutriment; to the similar material which is being presented or becoming adherent, the name of quasi-nutriment; and to everything else—that is, contained in the stomach and veins—the name of destined nutriment.

12 It is quite clear, therefore, that nutrition must necessarily be a process of assimilation of that which is nourishing to that which is being nourished. Some, however, say that this assimilation does not occur in reality, but is merely apparent; these are the people who think that Nature is not artistic, that she does not show forethought for the animal's welfare, and that she has absolutely no native powers whereby she alters some substances, attracts others, and discharges others. Now, speaking generally, there have arisen the following two sects in medicine and philosophy among those who have made any definite pronouncement regarding Nature. I speak, of course, of such of them as know what they are talking about, and who realize the logical sequence of their hypotheses, and stand by them; as for those who cannot understand even this, but who simply talk any nonsense that comes to their tongues, and who do not remain definitely attached either to one sect or the other—such people are not even worth mentioning. What, then, are these sects, and what are the logical consequences of their hypotheses? The one class supposes that all substance which is subject to genesis and destruction is at once continuous and susceptible of alteration.

The other school assumes substance to be unchangeable, unalterable, and subdivided into fine particles, which are separated from one another by empty spaces. All people, therefore, who can appreciate the logical sequence of an hypothesis hold that, according to the second teaching, there does not exist any substance or faculty peculiar either to Nature or to Soul, but that these result from the way in which the primary corpuscles, which are unaffected by change, come together. According to the first-mentioned teaching, on the other hand, Nature is not posterior to the corpuscles, but is a long way prior to them and older that they; and therefore in their view it is Nature which puts together the bodies both of plants and animals; and this she does by virtue of certain faculties which she possesses—these being, on the one hand, attractive and assimilative of what is appropriate, and, on the other, of what is foreign. Further, she skillfully molds everything during the stage of genesis; and she also provides for the creatures after birth, employing here other faculties again, namely, one of affection and forethought for offspring, and one of sociability and friendship for kindred. According to the other school, none of these things exist in the natures [of living things], nor is there in the soul any original innate idea, whether of agreement or difference, of separation or synthesis, of justice or injustice, of the beautiful or ugly; all such things, they say, arise in us from sensation and through sensation, and animals are steered by certain images and memories.

Some of these people have even expressly declared that the soul possesses no reasoning faculty, but that we are led like cattle by the impression of our senses, and are unable to refuse or dissent from anything. In their view, obviously, courage, wisdom, temperance, and self-control are all mere nonsense, we do not love either each other or our offspring, nor do the gods care anything for us. This school also despises dreams, birds, omens, and the whole of astrology, subjects with which we have dealt at a greater length in another work, in which we discuss the views of Asclepiades the physician. Those who wish to do so may familiarize themselves with these arguments, and they may also consider at this point which of the two roads lying before us is the better one to take. Hippocrates took the first-mentioned. According to this teaching, substance is one and is subject to alteration; there is a consensus in the movements of air and fluid throughout the whole body; Nature acts throughout in an artistic and equitable manner, having certain faculties, by virtue of which each part of the body draws to itself the juice which is proper to it, and, having done so, attaches it to every portion of itself, and completely assimilates it; while such part of the juice as has not been mastered, and is not capable of undergoing complete alteration and being assimilated to the part which is being nourished, is got rid of by yet another (an expulsive) faculty.

13 Now the extent of exactitude and truth in the doctrines of Hippocrates may be gauged, not merely from the way in which his opponents are at variance with obvious facts, but also from the various subjects of natural research themselves—the functions of animals, and the rest. For those people who do not believe that there exists in any part of the animal a faculty for attracting its own special quality are compelled repeatedly to deny obvious facts. For instance, Asclepiades, the physician, did this in the case of the kidneys. That these are organs for secreting [separating out] the urine, was the belief not only of Hippocrates, Diocles, Erasistratus, Praxagoras, and all the other physicians of eminence, but practically every butcher is aware of this, from the fact that he daily observes both the position of the kidneys and the duct (termed the ureter) which runs from each kidney into the bladder, and from this arrangement he infers their characteristic use and faculty. But, even leaving the butchers aside, all people who suffer either from frequent dysuria or from retention of urine call themselves "nephritics," when they feel pain in the loins and pass sandy matter in their water.

I do not suppose that Asclepiades ever saw a stone which had been passed by one of these sufferers or observed that this was preceded by a sharp pain in the region between the kidneys and the bladder as the stone traversed the ureter, or that, when the stone was passed, both the pain and the retention at once ceased. It is worth while, then, learning how his theory account for the presence of urine in the bladder, and one is forced to marvel at the ingenuity of a man who puts aside these broad, clearly visible routes, and postulates others which are narrow, invisible—indeed, entirely imperceptible. His view, in fact, is that the fluid which we drink passes into the bladder by being resolved into vapors, and that, when these have again been condensed, it thus regains its previous form, and turns from vapor into fluid. He simply looks upon the bladder as a sponge or a piece of wool, and not as the perfectly compact and impervious body that it is, with two very strong coats. For if we say that the vapors pass through these coats, why should they not pass through the peritoneum and the diaphragm, thus filling the whole abdominal cavity and thorax with water? "But," says he, "of course the peritoneal coat is more impervious than the bladder, and this is why it keeps out the vapors, while the bladder admits them." Yet if he had ever practiced anatomy, he might have known that the outer coat of the bladder springs from the peritoneum and is essentially the same as it, and that the inner coat, which is peculiar to the bladder, is more than twice as thick as the former. Perhaps, however, it is not the thickness or thinness of the coats, but the situation of the bladder, which is the reason for the vapours being carried into it? On the contrary, even if it were probable for every other reason that the vapours accumulate there, yet the situation of the bladder would be enough in itself to prevent this. For the bladder is situated below, whereas vapours have a natural tendency to rise upwards; thus they would fill all the region of the thorax and lungs long before they came to the bladder.

But why do I mention the situation of the bladder, peritoneum, and thorax? For surely, when the vapours have passed through the coats of the stomach and intestines, it is in the space between these and the peritoneum that they will collect and become liquefied (just as in dropsical subjects it is in this region that most of the water gathers). Otherwise the vapours must necessarily pass straight forward through everything which in any way comes into contact with them, and will never come to a standstill. But, if this be assumed, then they will traverse not merely the peritoneum but also the epigastrium, and will become dispersed into the surrounding air; otherwise they will certainly collect under the skin. Even these considerations, however, our present-day Asclepiadeans attempt to answer, despite the fact that they always get soundly laughed at by all who happen to be present at their disputations on these subjects—so difficult an evil to get rid of is this sectarian partizanship, so excessively resistant to all cleansing process, harder to heal than any itch! Thus, one of our Sophists who is a thoroughly hardened disputer and as skilful a master of language as there ever was, once got into a discussion with me on this subject; so far from being put out of countenance by any of the above-mentioned considerations, he even expressed his surprise that I should try to overturn obvious facts by ridiculous arguments! "For," said he, "one may clearly observe any day in the case of the bladder, that, if one fills it with water or air and then ties up its neck and squeezes it all round, it does not let anything out at any point, but accurately retains all its contents. And surely," said he, "if there were any large and perceptible channels coming into it from the kidneys the liquid would run out through these when the bladder was squeezed, in the same way that it entered?" Having abruptly made these and similar remarks in precise and clear tones, he concluded by jumping up and departing—leaving me as though I were quite incapable of finding any plausible answer!

The fact is that those who are enslaved to their sects are not merely devoid of all sound knowledge, but they will not even stop to learn! Instead of listening, as they ought, to the reason why liquid can enter the bladder through the ureters, but is unable to go back again the same way,—instead of admiring Nature's artistic skill—they refuse to learn; they even go so far as to scoff, and maintain that the kidneys, as well as many other things, have been made by Nature for no purpose! And some of them who had allowed themselves to be shown the ureters coming from the kidneys and becoming implanted in the bladder, even had the audacity to say that these also existed for no purpose; and others said that they were spermatic ducts, and that this was why they were inserted into the neck of the bladder and not into its cavity. When, therefore, we had demonstrated to them the real spermatic ducts entering the neck of the bladder lower down than the ureters, we supposed that, if we had not done so before, we would now at least draw them away from their false assumptions, and convert them forthwith to the opposite view. But even this they presumed to dispute, and said that it was not to be wondered at that the semen should remain longer in these latter ducts, these being more constricted, and that it should flow quickly down the ducts which came from the kidneys, seeing that these were well dilated. We were, therefore, further compelled to show them in a still living animal, the urine plainly running out through the ureters into the bladder; even thus we hardly hoped to check their nonsensical talk.

Now the method of demonstration is as follows. One has to divide the peritoneum in front of the ureters, then secure these with ligatures, and next, having bandaged up the animal, let him go (for he will not continue to urinate). After this one loosens the external bandages and shows the bladder empty and the ureters quite full and distended—in fact almost on the point of rupturing; on removing the ligature from them, one then plainly sees the bladder becoming filled with urine. When this has been made quite clear, then, before the animal urinates, one has to tie a ligature round his penis and then to squeeze the bladder all over; still nothing goes back through the ureters to the kidneys. Here, then, it becomes obvious that not only in a dead animal, but in one which is still living, the ureters are prevented from receiving back the urine from the bladder. These observations having been made, one now loosens the ligature from the animal's penis and allows him to urinate, then again ligatures one of the ureters and leaves the other to discharge into the bladder. Allowing, then, some time to elapse, one now demonstrates that the ureter which was ligatured is obviously full and distended on the side next to the kidneys, while the other one—that from which the ligature had been taken—is itself flaccid, but has filled the bladder with urine. Then, again, one must divide the full ureter, and demonstrate how the urine spurts out of it, like blood in the operation of vene-section; and after this one cuts through the other one also, and both being thus divided, one bandages up the animal externally.

Then when enough time seems to have elapsed, one takes off the bandages; the bladder will now be found empty, and the whole region between the intestines and the peritoneum full of urine, as if the animal were suffering from dropsy. Now, if anyone will but test this for himself on an animal, I think he will strongly condemn the rashness of Asclepiades, and if he learns the reason why nothing regurgitates from the bladder into the ureters, I think he will be persuaded by this also of the forethought and art shown by Nature in relation to animals. Now Hippocrates, who was the first known to us of all those who have been both physicians and philosophers in as much as he was the first to recognize what Nature effects, expresses his admiration of her, and is constantly singing her praises and calling her "just." Alone, he says, she suffices for the animal in every respect, performing of her accord and without any teaching all that is required. Being such, she has, as he supposes, certain faculties, one attractive of what is appropriate, and another eliminative of what is foreign, and she nourishes the animal, makes it grow, and expels its diseases by crisis. Therefore he says that there is in our bodies a concordance in the movements of air and fluid, and that everything is in sympathy. According to Asclepiades, however, nothing is naturally in sympathy with anything else, all substance being divided and broken up into inharmonious elements and absurd "molecules." Necessarily, then, besides making countless other statements in opposition to plain fact, he was ignorant of Nature's faculties, both that attracting what is appropriate, and that expelling what is foreign.

Thus he invented some wretched nonsense to explain blood-production and anadosis, and, being utterly unable to find anything to say regarding the clearing-out of the superfluities, he did not hesitate to join issue with obvious facts, and, in this matter of urinary secretion, to deprive both the kidneys and the ureters of their activity, by assuming that there were certain invisible channels opening into the bladder. It was, of course, a grand and impressive thing to do, to mistrust the obvious, and to pin one's faith in things which could not be seen! Also, in the matter of the yellow bile, he makes an even grander and more spirited venture; for he says this is actually generated in the bile-ducts, not merely separated out. How comes it, then, that in cases of jaundice two things happen at the same time—that the dejections contain absolutely no bile, and that the whole body becomes full of it? He is forced here again to talk nonsense, just as he did in regard to the urine. He also talks no less nonsense about the black bile and the spleen, not understanding what was said by Hippocrates; and he attempts in stupid—I might say insane—language, to contradict what he knows nothing about. And what profit did he derive from these opinions from the point of view of treatment? He neither was able to cure a kidney ailment, nor jaundice, nor a disease of black bile, nor would he agree with the view held not merely by Hippocrates but by all men regarding drugs—that some of them purge away yellow bile, and others black, some again phlegm, and others the thin and watery superfluity; he held that all the substances evacuated were produced by the drugs themselves, just as yellow bile is produced by the biliary passages! It matters nothing, according to this extraordinary man, whether we give a hydragogue or a cholagogue in a case of dropsy, for these all equally purge and dissolve the body, and produce a solution having such and such an appearance, which did not exist as such before! Must we not, therefore, suppose he was either mad, or entirely unacquainted with practical medicine? For who does not know that if a drug for attracting phlegm be given in a case of jaundice it will not even evacuate four cyathi of phlegm?

Similarly, also if one of the hydragogues be given. A cholagogue, on the other hand, clears away a great quantity of bile, and the skin of patients so treated at once becomes clear. I myself have, in many cases, after treating the liver condition, then removed the disease by means of a single purgation; whereas, if one had employed a drug for removing phlegm one would have done no good. Nor is Hippocrates the only one who knows this to be so, whilst those who take experience alone as their starting-point know otherwise; they, as well as all physicians who are trained in the practice of medicine, are of this opinion. Asclepiades, however, is an exception; he would hold it a betrayal of his assumed "elements" to confess the truth about such matters. For if a single drug were to be discovered which attracted such and such a humour only, there would obviously be danger of the opinion gaining ground that there is in every body a faculty which attracts its own particular quality. He therefore says that safflower, the Cnidian berry, and Hippophaes, do not draw phlegm from the body, but actually make it. Moreover, he holds that the flower and scales of bronze, and burnt bronze itself, and germander, and wild mastich dissolve the body into water, and that dropsical patients derive benefit from these substances, not because they are purged by them, but because they are rid of substances which actually help to increase the disease; for, if the medicine does not evacuate the dropsical fluid contained in the body, but generates it, it aggravates the condition further.

Moreover, scammony, according to the Asclepiadean argument, not only fails to evacuate the bile from the bodies of jaundiced subjects, but actually turns the useful blood into bile, and dissolves the body; in fact it does all manner of evil and increases the disease. And yet this drug may be clearly seen to do good to numbers of people! "Yes," says he, "they derive benefit certainly, but merely in proportion to the evacuation." . . . But if you give these cases a drug which draws off phlegm they will not be benefited. This is so obvious that even those who make experience alone their starting-point are aware of it; and these people make it a cardinal point of their teaching to trust to no arguments, but only to what can be clearly seen. In this, then, they show good sense; whereas Asclepiades goes far astray in bidding us distrust our senses where obvious facts plainly overturn his hypotheses. Much better would it have been for him not to assail obvious facts, but rather to devote himself entirely to these. Is it, then, these facts only which are plainly irreconcilable with the views of Asclepiades? Is not also the fact that in summer yellow bile is evacuated in greater quantity by the same drugs, and in winter phlegm, and that in a young man more bile is evacuated, and in an old man more phlegm? Obviously each drug attracts something which already exists, and does not generate something previously non-existent. Thus if you give in the summer season a drug which attracts phlegm to a young man of a lean and warm habit, who has lived neither idly nor too luxuriously, you will with great difficulty evacuate a very small quantity of this humour, and you will do the man the utmost harm. On the other hand, if you give him a cholagogue, you will produce an abundant evacuation and not injure him at all. Do we still, then, disbelieve that each drug attracts that humour which is proper to it? Possibly the adherents of Asclepiades will assent to this—or rather, they will—not possibly, but certainly—declare that they disbelieve it, lest they should betray their darling prejudices.

14 Let us pass on, then, again to another piece of nonsense; for the sophists do not allow one to engage in enquiries that are of any worth, albeit there are many such; they compel one to spend one's time in dissipating the fallacious arguments which they bring forward. What, then, is this piece of nonsense? It has to do with the famous and far-renowned stone which draws iron [the lodestone]. It might be thought that this would draw their minds to a belief that there are in all bodies certain faculties by which they attract their own proper qualities. Now Epicurus, despite the fact that he employs in his *Physics* elements similar to those of Asclepiades, yet allows that iron is attracted by the lodestone, and chaff by amber. He even tries to give the cause of the phenomenon. His view is that the atoms which flow from the stone are related in shape to those flowing from the iron, and so they become easily interlocked with one another; thus it is that, after colliding with each of the two compact masses (the stone and the iron) they then rebound into the middle and so become entangled with each other, and draw the iron after them. So far, then, as his hypotheses regarding causation go, he is perfectly unconvincing; nevertheless, he does grant that there is an attraction. Further, he says that it is on similar principles that there occur in the bodies of animals the dispersal of nutriment and the discharge of waste matters, as also the actions of cathartic drugs. Asclepiades, however, who viewed with suspicion the incredible character of the cause mentioned, and who saw no other credible cause on the basis of his supposed elements, shamelessly had recourse to the statement that nothing is in any way attracted by anything else.

Now, if he was dissatisfied with what Epicurus said, and had nothing better to say himself, he ought to have refrained from making hypotheses, and should have said that Nature is a constructive artist and that the substance of things is always tending towards unity and also towards alteration because its own parts act upon and are acted upon by one another. For, if he had assumed this, it would not have been difficult to allow that this constructive Nature has powers which attract appropriate and expel alien matter. For in no other way could she be constructive, preservative of the animal, and eliminative of its diseases, unless it be allowed that she conserves what is appropriate and discharges what is foreign. But in this matter, too, Asclepiades realized the logical sequence of the principles he had assumed; he showed no scruples, however, in opposing plain fact; he joins issue in this matter also, not merely with all physicians, but with everyone else, and maintains that there is no such thing as a crisis, or critical day, and that Nature does absolutely nothing for the preservation of the animal. For his constant aim is to follow out logical consequences and to upset obvious fact, in this respect being opposed to Epicurus; for the latter always stated the observed fact, although he gives an ineffective explanation of it. For, that these small corpuscles belonging to the lodestone rebound, and become entangled with other similar particles of the iron, and that then, by means of this entanglement (which cannot be seen anywhere) such a heavy substance as iron is attracted—I fail to understand how anybody could believe this. Even if we admit this, the same principle will not explain the fact that, when the iron has another piece brought in contact with it, this becomes attached to it. For what are we to say? That, forsooth, some of the particles that flow from the lodestone collide with the iron and then rebound back, and that it is by these that the iron becomes suspended? that others penetrate into it, and rapidly pass through it by way of its empty channels? that these then collide with the second piece of iron and are not able to penetrate it although they penetrated the first piece? and that they then course back to the first piece, and produce entanglements like the former ones? The hypothesis here becomes clearly refuted by its absurdity.

As a matter of fact, I have seen five writing-stylets of iron attached to one another in a line, only the first one being in contact with the lodestone, and the power being transmitted through it to the others. Moreover, it cannot be said that if you bring a second stylet into contact with the lower end of the first, it becomes held, attached, and suspended, whereas, if you apply it to any other part of the side it does not become attached. For the power of the lodestone is distributed in all directions; it merely needs to be in contact with the first stylet at any point; from this stylet again the power flows, as quick as a thought, all through the second, and from that again to the third. Now, if you imagine a small lodestone hanging in a house, and in contact with it all round a large number of pieces of iron, from them again others, and so on,—all these pieces of iron must surely become filled with the corpuscles which emanate from the stone; therefore, this first little stone is likely to become dissipated by disintegrating into these emanations. Further, even if there be no iron in contact with it, it still disperses into the air, particularly if this be also warm.

"Yes," says Epicurus, "but these corpuscles must be looked on as exceedingly small, so that some of them are a ten-thousandth part of the size of the very smallest particles carried in the air." Then do you venture to say that so great a weight of iron can be suspended by such small bodies? If each of them is a ten-thousandth part as large as the dust particles which are borne in the atmosphere, how big must we suppose the hook-like extremities by which they interlock with each other to be? For of course this is quite the smallest portion of the whole particle. Then, again, when a small body becomes entangled with another small body, or when a body in motion becomes entangled with another also in motion, they do not rebound at once. For, further, there will of course be others which break in upon them from above, from below, from front and rear, from right and left, and which shake and agitate them and never let them rest.

Moreover, we must perforce suppose that each of these small bodies has a large number of these hook-like extremities. For by one it attaches itself to its neighbours, by another—the topmost one—to the lodestone, and by the bottom one to the iron. For if it were attached to the stone above and not interlocked with the iron below, this would be of no use. Thus, the upper part of the superior extremity must hang from the lodestone, and the iron must be attached to the lower end of the inferior extremity; and, since they interlock with each other by their sides as well, they must, of course, have hooks there too. Keep in mind also, above everything, what small bodies these are which possess all these different kinds of outgrowths. Still more, remember how, in order that the second piece of iron may become attached to the first, the third to the second, and to that the fourth, these absurd little particles must both penetrate the passages in the first piece of iron and at the same time rebound from the piece coming next in the series, although this second piece is naturally in every way similar to the first. Such an hypothesis, once again, is certainly not lacking in audacity; in fact, to tell the truth, it is far more shameless than the previous ones; according to it, when five similar pieces of iron are arranged in a line, the particles of the lodestone which easily traverse the first piece of iron rebound from the second, and do not pass readily through it in the same way. Indeed, it is nonsense, whichever alternative is adopted. For, if they do rebound, how then do they pass through into the third piece? And if they do not rebound, how does the second piece become suspended to the first? For Epicurus himself looked on the rebound as the active agent in attraction. But, as I have said, one is driven to talk nonsense whenever one gets into discussion with such men.

Having, therefore, given a concise and summary statement of the matter, I wish to be done with it.

For if one diligently familiarizes oneself with the writings of Asclepiades, one will see clearly their logical dependence on his first principles, but also their disagreement with observed facts. Thus, Epicurus, in his desire to adhere to the facts, cuts an awkward figure by aspiring to show that these agree with his principles, whereas Asclepiades safeguards the sequence of principles, but pays no attention to the obvious fact. Whoever, therefore, wishes to expose the absurdity of these hypotheses, must, if the argument be in answer to Asclepiades, keep in mind his disagreement with observed fact; or if in answer to Epicurus, his discordance with his principles. Almost all the other sects depending on similar principles are now entirely extinct, while these alone maintain a respectable existence still. Yet the tenets of Asclepiades have been unanswerably confuted by Menodotus the Empiricist, who draws his attention to their opposition to phenomena and to each other; and, again, those of Epicurus have been confuted by Asclepiades, who adhered always to logical sequence, about which Epicurus evidently cares little. Now people of the present day do not begin by getting a clear comprehension of these sects, as well as of the better ones, thereafter devoting a long time to judging and testing the true and false in each of them; despite their ignorance, they style themselves, some "physicians" and others "philosophers."

No wonder, then, that they honour the false equally with the true. For everyone becomes like the first teacher that he comes across, without waiting to learn anything from anybody else. And there are some of them, who, even if they meet with more than one teacher, are yet so unintelligent and slow-witted that even by the time they have reached old age they are still incapable of understanding the steps of an argument. . . . In the old days such people used to be set to menial tasks. . . . What will be the end of it God knows! Now, we usually refrain from arguing with people whose principles are wrong from the outset. Still, having been compelled by the natural course of events to enter into some kind of a discussion with them, we must add this further to what was said—that it is not only cathartic drugs which naturally attract their special qualities, but also those which remove thorns and the points of arrows such as sometimes become deeply embedded in the flesh. Those drugs also which draw out animal poisons or poisons applied to arrows all show the same faculty as does the lodestone. Thus, I myself have seen a thorn which was embedded in a young man's foot fail to come out when we exerted forcible traction with our fingers, and yet come away painlessly and rapidly on the application of a medicament.

Yet even to this some people will object, asserting that when the inflammation is dispersed from the part the thorn comes away of itself, without being pulled out by anything. But these people seem, in the first place, to be unaware that there are certain drugs for drawing out inflammation and different ones for drawing out embedded substances; and surely if it was on the cessation of an inflammation that the abnormal matters were expelled, then all drugs which disperse inflammations ought ipso facto to possess the power of extracting these substances as well. And secondly, these people seem to be unaware of a still more surprising fact, namely, that not merely do certain medicaments draw out thorns and others poisons, but that of the latter there are some which attract the poison of the viper, others that of the sting-ray, and others that of some other animal; we can, in fact, plainly observe these poisons deposited on the medicaments. Here, then, we must praise Epicurus for the respect he shows towards obvious facts, but find fault with his views as to causation. For how can it be otherwise than extremely foolish to suppose that a thorn which we failed to remove by digital traction could be drawn out by these minute particles? Have we now, therefore, convinced ourselves that everything which exists possesses a faculty by which it attracts its proper quality, and that some things do this more, and some less? Or shall we also furnish our argument with the illustration afforded by corn? For those who refuse to admit that anything is attracted by anything else, will, I imagine, be here proved more ignorant regarding Nature than the very peasants. When, for my own part, I first learned of what happens, I was surprised, and felt anxious to see it with my own eyes. Afterwards, when experience also had confirmed its truth, I sought long among the various sects for an explanation, and, with the exception of that which gave the first place to attraction, I could find none which even approached plausibility, all the others being ridiculous and obviously quite untenable.

What happens, then, is the following. When our peasants are bringing corn from the country into the city in wagons, and wish to filch some away without being detected, they fill earthen jars with water and stand them among the corn; the corn then draws the moisture into itself through the jar and acquires additional bulk and weight, but the fact is never detected by the onlookers unless someone who knew about the trick before makes a more careful inspection. Yet, if you care to set down the same vessel in the very hot sun, you will find the daily loss to be very little indeed. Thus corn has a greater power than extreme solar heat of drawing to itself the moisture in its neighbourhood. Thus the theory that the water is carried towards the rarefied part of the air surrounding us (particularly when that is distinctly warm) is utter nonsense; for although it is much more rarefied there than it is amongst the corn, yet it does not take up a tenth part of the moisture which the corn does.

15 Since, then, we have talked sufficient nonsense—not willingly, but because we were forced, as the proverb says, "to behave madly among madmen"—let us return again to the subject of urinary secretion. Here let us forget the absurdities of Asclepiades, and, in company with those who are persuaded that the urine does pass through the kidneys, let us consider what is the character of this function. For, most assuredly, either the urine is conveyed by its own motion to the kidneys, considering this the better course (as do we when we go off to market!), or, if this be impossible, then some other reason for its conveyance must be found. What, then, is this? If we are not going to grant the kidneys a faculty for attracting this particular quality, as Hippocrates held, we shall discover no other reason. For, surely everyone sees that either the kidneys must attract the urine, or the veins must propel it—if, that is, it does not move of itself. But if the veins did exert a propulsive action when they contract, they would squeeze out into the kidneys not merely the urine, but along with it the whole of the blood which they contain. And if this is impossible, as we shall show, the remaining explanation is that the kidneys do exert traction. And how is propulsion by the veins impossible? The situation of the kidneys is against it. They do not occupy a position beneath the hollow vein [vena cava] as does the sieve-like [ethmoid] passage in the nose and palate in relation to the surplus matter from the brain; they are situated on both sides of it. Besides, if the kidneys are like sieves, and readily let the thinner serous [whey-like] portion through, and keep out the thicker portion, then the whole of the blood contained in the vena cava must go to them, just as the whole of wine is thrown into the filters. Further, the example of milk being made into cheese will show clearly what I mean. For this, too, although it is all thrown into the wicker strainers, does not all percolate through; such part of it as is too fine in proportion to the width of the meshes passes downwards, and this is called whey [serum]; the remaining thick portion which is destined to become cheese cannot get down, since the pores of the strainers will not admit it.

Thus it is that, if the blood-serum has similarly to percolate through the kidneys, the whole of the blood must come to them, and not merely one part of it. What, then, is the appearance as found on dissection? One division of the vena cava is carried upwards to the heart, and the other mounts upon the spine and extends along its whole length as far as the legs; thus one division does not even come near the kidneys, while the other approaches them but is certainly not inserted into them. Now, if the blood were destined to be purified by them as if they were sieves, the whole of it would have to fall into them, the thin part being and the thick part retained above. But, as a matter of fact, this is not so. For the kidneys lie on either side of the vena cava. They therefore do not act like sieves, filtering fluid sent to them by the vena cava, and themselves contributing no force. They obviously exert traction; for this is the remaining alternative. How, then, do they exert this traction?

If, as Epicurus thinks, all attraction takes place by virtue of the rebounds and entanglements of atoms, it would be certainly better to maintain that the kidneys have no attractive action at all; for his theory, when examined, would be found as it stands to be much more ridiculous even than the theory of the lodestone, mentioned a little while ago. Attraction occurs in the way that Hippocrates laid down; this will be stated more clearly as the discussion proceeds; for the present our task is not to demonstrate this, but to point out that no other cause of the secretion of urine can be given except that of attraction by the kidneys, and that this attraction does not take place in the way imagined by people who do not allow Nature a faculty of her own. For if it be granted that there is any attractive faculty at all in those things which are governed by Nature, a person who attempted to say anything else about the absorption of nutriment would be considered a fool.

16 Now, while Erasistratus for some reason replied at great length to certain other foolish doctrines, he entirely passed over the view held by Hippocrates, not even thinking it worth while to mention it, as he did in his work *On Deglutition;* in that work, as may be seen, he did go so far as at least to make mention of the word attraction, writing somewhat as follows: *Now, the stomach does not appear to exercise any attraction.* But when he is dealing with anadosis he does not mention the Hippocratic view even to the extent of a single syllable. Yet we should have been satisfied if he had even merely written this: "Hippocrates lies in saying 'The flesh attracts both from the stomach and from without,' for it cannot attract either from the stomach or from without." Or if he had thought it worth while to state that Hippocrates was wrong in criticizing the weakness of the neck of the uterus, "seeing that the orifice of the uterus has no power of attracting semen," or if he [Erasistratus] had thought proper to write any other similar opinion, then we in our turn would have defended ourselves in the following terms: "My good sir, do not run us down in this rhetorical fashion without some proof; state some definite objection to our view, in order that either you may convince us by a brilliant refutation of the ancient doctrine, or that, on the other hand, we may convert you from your ignorance." Yet why do I say "rhetorical"? For we too are not to suppose that when certain rhetoricians pour ridicule upon that which they are quite incapable of refuting, without any attempt at argument, their words are really thereby constituted rhetoric. For rhetoric proceeds by persuasive reasoning; words without reasoning are buffoonery rather than rhetoric. Therefore, the reply of Erasistratus in his treatise *On Deglutition* was neither rhetoric nor logic. For what is it that he says? *Now, the stomach does not appear to exercise any traction.*

Let us testify against him in return, and set our argument beside his in the same form. Now, there appears to be no peristalsis of the gullet. "And how does this appear?" one of his adherents may perchance ask. "For is it not indicative of peristalsis that always when the upper parts of the gullet contract the lower parts dilate?" Again, then, we say, "And in what way does the attraction of the stomach not appear?" Now, if he would but be sensible and recognize that this phenomenon is not more indicative of the one than the of the other view, but that it applies equally to both, we should then show him without further delay the proper way to the discovery of truth. We will, however, speak about the stomach again. And the dispersal of nutriment [anadosis] need not make us have recourse to the theory regarding the natural tendency of a vacuum to become refilled, when once we have granted the attractive faculty to the kidneys. Now, although Erasistratus knew that this faculty most certainly existed, he neither mentioned it nor denied it, nor did he make any statement as to his views on the secretion of urine. Why did he give notice at the very beginning of his *General Principles* that he was going to speak about natural activities—firstly what they are, how they take place, and in what situations—and then, in the case of urinary secretion, declared that this took place through the kidneys, but left out its method of occurrence? It must, then, have been for no purpose that he told us how digestion occurs, or spends time upon the secretion of biliary superfluities; for in these cases also it would have been sufficient to have named the parts through which the function takes place, and to have omitted the method.

On the contrary, in these cases he was able to tell us not merely through what organs, but also in what way it occurs—as he also did, I think, in the case of anadosis; for he was not satisfied with saying that this took place through the veins, but he also considered fully the method, which he held to be from the tendency of a vacuum to become refilled. Concerning the secretion of urine, however, he writes that this occurs through the kidneys, but does not add in what way it occurs. I do not think he could say that this was from the tendency of matter to fill a vacuum, for, if this were so, nobody would have ever died of retention of urine, since no more can flow into a vacuum than has run out. For, if no other factor comes into operation save only this tendency by which a vacuum becomes refilled, no more could ever flow in than had been evacuated. Nor, could he suggest any other plausible cause, such, for example, as that of nutriment by the stomach which occurs in the process of anadosis; this had been entirely disproved in the case of blood in the vena cava; it is excluded, not merely owing to the long distance, but also from the fact that the overlying heart, at each diastole, robs the vena cava by violence of a considerable quantity of blood. In relation to the lower part of the vena cava there would still remain, solitary and abandoned, the specious theory concerning the filling of a vacuum. This, however, is deprived of plausibility by the fact that people die of retention of urine, and also, no less, by the situation of the kidneys. For, if the whole of the blood were carried to the kidneys, one might properly maintain that it all undergoes purification there.

But, as a matter of fact, the whole of it does not go to them, but only so much as can be contained in the veins going to the kidneys; this portion only, therefore, will be purified. Further, the thin serous part of this will pass through the kidneys as if through a sieve, while the thick sanguineous portion remaining in the veins will obstruct the blood flowing in from behind; this will first, therefore, have to run back to the vena cava, and so to empty the veins going to the kidneys; these veins will no longer be able to conduct a second quantity of unpurified blood to the kidneys—occupied as they are by the blood which had preceded, there is no passage left. What power have we, then, which will draw back the purified blood from the kidneys? And what power, in the next place, will bid this blood retire to the lower part of the vena cava, and will enjoin on another quantity coming from above not to proceed downwards before turning off into the kidneys? Now Erasistratus realized that all these ideas were open to many objections, and he could only find one idea which held good in all respects—namely, that of attraction.

Since, therefore, he did not wish either to get into difficulties or to mention the view of Hippocrates, he deemed it better to say nothing at all as to the manner in which secretion occurs. But even if he kept silence, I am not going to do so. For I know that if one passes over the Hippocratic view and makes some other pronouncement about the function of the kidneys, one cannot fall to make oneself utterly ridiculous. It was for this reason that Erasistratus kept silence and Asclepiades lied; they are like slaves who have had plenty to say in the early part of their career, and have managed by excessive rascality to escape many and frequent accusations, but who, later, when caught in the act of thieving, cannot find any excuse; the more modest one then keeps silence, as though thunderstruck, whilst the more shameless continues to hide the missing article beneath his arm and denies on oath that he has ever seen it. For it was in this way also that Asclepiades, when all subtle excuses had failed him and there was no longer any room for nonsense about *conveyance towards the rarefied part [of the air]*, and when it was impossible without incurring the greatest derision to say that this superfluity [i.e. the urine] is generated by the kidneys as is bile by the canals in the liver—he, then, I say, clearly lied when he swore that the urine does not reach the kidneys, and maintained that it passes, in the form of vapour, straight from the region of the vena cava, to collect in the bladder. Like slaves, then, caught in the act of stealing, these two are quite bewildered, and while the one says nothing, the other indulges in shameless lying.

17 Now such of the younger men as have dignified themselves with the names of these two authorities by taking the appellations "Erasistrateans" or "Asclepiadeans" are like the *Davi* and *Getae*—the slaves introduced by the excellent Menander into his comedies. As these slaves held that they had done nothing fine unless they had cheated their masters three times, so also the men I am discussing have taken their time over the construction of impudent sophisms, the one party striving to prevent the lies of Asclepiades from ever being refuted, and the other saying stupidly what Erasistratus had the sense to keep silence about. But enough about the Asclepiadeans. The Erasistrateans, in attempting to say how the kidneys let the urine through, will do anything or suffer anything or try any shift in order to find some plausible explanation which does not demand the principle of attraction. Now those near the times of Erasistratus maintain that the parts above the kidneys receive pure blood, whilst the watery residue, being heavy, tends to run downwards; that this, after percolating through the kidneys themselves, is thus rendered serviceable, and is sent, as blood, to all the parts below the kidneys. For a certain period at least this view also found favour and flourished, and was held to be true; after a time, however, it became suspect to the Erasistrateans themselves, and at last they abandoned it. For apparently the following two points were assumed, neither of which is conceded by anyone, nor is even capable of being proved.

The first is the heaviness of the serous fluid, which was said to be produced in the vena cava, and which did not exist, apparently, at the beginning, when this fluid was being carried up from the stomach to the liver. Why, then, did it not at once run downwards when it was in these situations? And if the watery fluid is so heavy, what plausibility can anyone find in the statement that it assists in the process of anadosis? In the second place there is this absurdity, that even if it be agreed that all the watery fluid does fall downwards, and only when it is in the vena cava, still it is difficult, or, rather, impossible, to say through what means it is going to fall into the kidneys, seeing that these are not situated below, but on either side of the vena cava, and that the vena cava is not inserted into them, but merely sends a branch into each of them, as it also does into all the other parts. What doctrine, then, took the place of this one when it was condemned? One which to me seems far more foolish than the first, although it also flourished at one time. For they say, that if oil be mixed with water and poured upon the ground, each will take a different route, the one flowing this way and the other that, and that, therefore, it is not surprising that the watery fluid runs into the kidneys, while the blood falls downwards along the vena cava. Now this doctrine also stands already condemned. For why, of the countless veins which spring from the vena cava, should blood flow into all the others, and the serous fluid be diverted to those going to the kidneys? They have not answered the question which was asked; they merely state what happens and imagine they have thereby assigned the reason. Once again, then (the third cup to the Saviour!), let us now speak of the worst doctrine of all, lately invented by Lycus of Macedonia, but which is popular owing to its novelty. This Lycus, then, maintains, as though uttering an oracle from the inner sanctuary, that urine is residual matter from the nutrition of the kidneys! Now, the amount of urine passed every day shows clearly that it is the whole of the fluid drunk which becomes urine, except for that which comes away with the dejections or passes off as sweat or insensible perspiration.

This is most easily recognized in winter in those who are doing no work but are carousing, especially if the wine be thin and diffusable; these people readily pass almost the same quantity as they drink. And that even Erasistratus was aware of this is known to those who have read the first book of his *General Principles*. Thus Lycus is speaking neither good Erasistratism, nor good Asclepiadism, far less good Hippocratism. He is, therefore, as the saying is, like a white crow, which cannot mix with the genuine crows owing to its colour, nor with the pigeons owing to its size. For all this, however, he is not to be disregarded; he may, perhaps, be stating some wonderful truth, unknown to any of his predecessors.

Now it is agreed that all parts which are undergoing nutrition produce a certain amount of residue, but it is neither agreed nor is it likely, that the kidneys alone, small bodies as they are, could hold four whole congii [about twelve quarts], and sometimes even more, of residual matter. For this surplus must necessarily be greater in quantity in each of the larger viscera; thus, for example, that of the lung, if it corresponds in amount to the size of the viscus, will obviously be many times more than in the kidneys, and thus the whole of the thorax will become filled, and the animal will be at once suffocated. But if it be said that the residual matter is equal in amount in each of the other parts, where are the bladders, one may ask, through which it is excreted? For, if the kidneys produce in drinkers three and sometimes four congii of superfluous matter, that of each of the other viscera will be much more, and thus an enormous barrel will be needed to contain the waste products of them all. Yet one often urinates practically the same quantity as one has drunk, which would show that the whole of what one drinks goes to the kidneys. Thus the author of this third piece of trickery would appear to have achieved nothing, but to have been at once detected, and there still remains the original difficulty which was insoluble by Erasistratus and by all others except Hippocrates. I dwell purposely on this topic, knowing well that nobody else has anything to say about the function of the kidneys, but that either we must prove more foolish than the very butchers if we do not agree that the urine passes through the kidneys; or, if one acknowledges this, that then one cannot possibly give any other reason for the secretion than the principle of attraction. Now, if the movement of urine does not depend on the tendency of a vacuum to become refilled, it is clear that neither does that of the blood nor that of the bile; or if that of these latter does so, then so also does that of the former. For they must all be accomplished in one and the same way, even according to Erasistratus himself. This matter, however, will be discussed more fully in the book following this.

BOOK II

1 In the previous book we demonstrated that not only Erasistratus, but also all others who would say anything to the purpose about urinary secretion, must acknowledge that the kidneys possess some faculty which attracts to them this particular quality existing in the urine. Besides this we drew attention to the fact that the urine is not carried through the kidneys into the bladder by one method, the blood into parts of the animal by another, and the yellow bile separated out on yet another principle. For when once there has been demonstrated in any one organ, the drawing, or so-called epispastic faculty, there is then no difficulty in transferring it to the rest. Certainly, Nature did not give a power such as this to the kidneys without giving it also to the vessels which abstract the biliary fluid, nor did she give it to the latter without also it to each of the other parts. And, assuredly, if this is true, we must marvel that Erasistratus should make statements concerning the delivery of nutriment from the food-canal which are so false as to be detected even by Asclepiades.

Now, Erasistratus considers it absolutely certain that, if anything flows from the veins, one of two things must happen: either a completely empty space will result, or the contiguous quantum of fluid will run in and take the place of that which has been evacuated. Asclepiades, however, holds that not one of two, but one of three things must be said to result in the emptied vessels: either there will be an entirely empty space, or the contiguous portion will flow in, or the vessel will contract. For whereas, in the case of reeds and tubes it is true to say that, if these be submerged in water, and are emptied of the air which they contain in their lumens, then either a completely empty space will be left, or the contiguous portion will move onwards; in the case of the veins this no longer holds, since their coats can collapse and so fall in upon the interior cavity. It may be seen, then, how false this hypothesis—by Zeus, I cannot call it a demonstration!—of Erasistratus is. And, from another point of view, even if it were true, it is superfluous, if the stomach has the power of compressing the veins, as he himself supposed, and the veins again of contracting upon their contents and propelling them forwards. For, apart from other considerations, no plethora would ever take place in the body, if delivery of nutriment resulted merely from the tendency of a vacuum to become refilled. Now, if the compression of the stomach becomes weaker the further it goes, and cannot reach to an indefinite distance, and if, therefore, there is need of some other mechanism to explain why the blood is conveyed in all directions, then the principle of the refilling of a vacuum may be looked on as a necessary addition; there will not, however, be a plethora in any of the parts coming after the liber, or, if there be, it will be in the region of the heart and lungs; for the heart alone of the parts which come after the liver draws the nutriment into its right ventricle, thereafter sending it through the arterial vein [what we now call the pulmonary artery] to the lungs (for Erasistratus himself will have it that, owing to the membranous excrescences, no other parts save the lungs receive nourishment from the heart).

If, however, in order to explain how plethora comes about, we suppose the force of compression by the stomach to persist indefinitely, we have no further need of the principle of the refilling of a vacuum, especially if we assume contraction of the veins in addition—as is, again, agreeable to Erasistratus himself.

2 Let me draw his attention, then, once again, even if he does not wish it, to the kidneys, and let me state that these confute in the very clearest manner such people as object to the principle of attraction. Nobody has ever said anything plausible, nor, as we previously showed, has anyone been able to discover, by any means, any other cause for the secretion of urine; we necessarily appear mad if we maintain that the urine passes into the kidneys in the form of vapor, and we certainly cut a poor figure when we talk about the tendency of a vacuum to become refilled; this idea is foolish in the case of blood, and impossible, nay, perfectly nonsensical, in the case of the urine. This, then, is one blunder made by those who dissociate themselves from the principle of attraction. Another is that which they make about the secretion of yellow bile. For in this case, too, it is not a fact that when the blood runs past the mouths [stomata] of the bile-ducts there will be a thorough separation out [secretion] of biliary waste-mater. "Well," say they, "let us suppose that it is not secreted but carried with the blood all over the body." But, you sapient folk, Erasistratus himself supposed that Nature took thought for the animals' future, and was workmanlike in her method; and at the same time he maintained that the biliary fluid was useless in every way for the animals. Now these two things are incompatible. For how could Nature be still looked on as exercising forethought for the animal when she allowed a noxious humour such as this to be carried off and distributed with the blood? . . .

This, however, is a small matter. I shall again point out here the greatest and most obvious error. For if the yellow bile adjusts itself to the narrower vessels and stomata, and the blood to the wider ones, for no other reason than that blood is thicker and bile thinner, and that the stomata of the veins are wider and those of the bile-ducts narrower, then it is clear that this watery and serous superfluity, too, will run out into the bile-ducts quicker than does the bile, exactly in proportion as it is thinner than the bile! How is it, then, that it does not run out? "Because," it may be said, "urine is thicker than bile!" This was what one of our Erasistrateans ventured to say, herein clearly disregarding the evidence of his senses, although he had trusted these in the case of the bile and blood. For, if it be that we are to look on bile as thinner than blood because it runs more, then, since the serous residue [blood-serum] passes through fine linen or lint or a sieve more easily even than does bile, by these tokens bile must also be thicker than the watery fluid. For here, again, there is no argument which will demonstrate that bile is thinner than the serous superfluities. But when a man shamelessly goes on using circumlocutions, and never acknowledges when he has had a fall, he is like the amateur wrestlers, who, when they have been overthrown by the experts and are lying on their backs on the ground, so far from recognizing their fall, actually seize their victorious adversaries by the necks and prevent them from getting away, thus supposing themselves to be the winners!

3 Thus, every hypothesis of channels as an explanation of natural functioning is perfect nonsense. For, if there were not an inborn faculty given by Nature to each one of the organs at the very beginning, then animals could not continue to live even for a few days, far less for the number of years which they actually do. For let us suppose they were under no guardianship, lacking in creative ingenuity and forethought; let us suppose they were steered only by material forces, and not by any special faculties (the one attracting what is proper to it, another rejecting what is foreign, and yet another causing alteration and adhesion of the matter destined to nourish it); if we suppose this, I am sure it would be ridiculous for us to discuss natural, or, still more, psychical, activities—or, in fact, life as a whole. For there is not a single animal which could live or endure for the shortest time if, possessing within itself so many different parts, it did not employ faculties which were attractive of what is appropriate, eliminative of what is foreign, and alterative of what is destined for nutrition.

On the other hand, if we have these faculties, we no longer need channels, little or big, resting on an unproven hypothesis, for explaining the secretion of urine and bile, and the conception of some favourable situation (in which point alone Erasistratus shows some common sense, since he does regard all the parts of the body as having been well and truly placed and shaped by Nature). But let us suppose he remained true to his own statement that Nature is "artistic"—this Nature which, at the beginning, well and truly shaped and disposed all the parts of the animal, and, after carrying out this function (for she left nothing undone), brought it forward to the light of day, endowed with certain faculties necessary for its very existence, and, thereafter, gradually increased it until it reached its due size. If he argued consistently on this principle, I fail to see how he can continue to refer natural functions to the smallness or largeness of canals, or to any other similarly absurd hypothesis. For this Nature which shapes and gradually adds to the parts is most certainly extended throughout their whole substance. Yes indeed, she shapes and nourishes and increases them through and through, not on the outside only. For Praxiteles and Phidias and all the other statuaries used merely to decorate their material on the outside, in so far as they were able to touch it; but its inner parts they left unembellished, unwrought, unaffected by art or forethought, since they were unable to penetrate therein and to reach and handle all portions of the material.

It is not so, however, with Nature. Every part of a bone she makes bone, every part of the flesh she makes flesh, and so with fat and all the rest; there is no part which she has not touched, elaborated, and embellished. Phidias, on the other hand, could not turn wax into ivory and gold, nor yet gold into wax: for each of these remains as it was at the commencement, and becomes a perfect statue simply by being clothed externally in a form and artificial shape. But Nature does not preserve the original character of any kind of matter; if she did so, then all parts of the animal would be blood—that blood, namely, which flows to the semen from the impregnated female and which is, so to speak, like the statuary's wax, a single uniform matter, subjected to the artificer. From this blood there arises no part of the animal which is as red and moist [as blood is], for bone, artery, vein, nerve, cartilage, fat, gland, membrane, and marrow are not blood, though they arise from it. I would then ask Erasistratus himself to inform me what the altering, coagulating, and shaping agent is. He would doubtless say, "Either Nature or the semen," meaning the same thing in both cases, but explaining it by different devices. For that which was previously semen, when it begins to procreate and to shape the animal, becomes, so to say, a special nature. For in the same way that Phidias possessed the faculties of his art even before touching his material, and then activated these in connection with this material (for every faculty remains inoperative in the absence of its proper material), so it is with the semen: its faculties it possessed from the beginning, while its activities it does not receive from its material, but it manifests them in connection therewith. And, of course, if it were to be overwhelmed with a great quantity of blood, it would perish, while if it were to be entirely deprived of blood it would remain inoperative and would not turn into a nature.

Therefore, in order that it may not perish, but may become a nature in place of semen, there must be an afflux to it of a little blood—or, rather, one should not say a little, but a quantity commensurate with that of the semen. What is it then that measures the quantity of this afflux? What prevents more from coming? What ensures against a deficiency? What is this third overseer of animal generation that we are to look for, which will furnish the semen with a due amount of blood? What would Erasistratus have said if he had been alive, and had been asked this question? Obviously, the semen itself. This, in fact, is the artificer analogous with Phidias, whilst the blood corresponds to the statuary's wax. Now, it is not for the wax to discover for itself how much of it is required; that is the business of Phidias. Accordingly the artificer will draw to itself as much blood as it needs. Here, however, we must pay attention and take care not unwittingly to credit the semen with reason and intelligence; if we were to do this, we would be making neither semen nor a nature, but an actual living animal. And if we retain these two principles—that of proportionate attraction and that of the non-participation of intelligence—we shall ascribe to the semen a faculty for attracting blood similar to that possessed by the lodestone for iron. Here, then, again, in the case of the semen, as in so many previous instances, we have been compelled to acknowledge some kind of attractive faculty. And what is the semen? Clearly the active principle of the animal, the material principle being the menstrual blood. Next, seeing that the active principle employs this faculty primarily, therefore, in order that any one of the things fashioned by it may come into existence, it [the principle] must necessarily be possessed of its own faculty. How, then, was Erasistratus unaware of it, if the primary function of the semen be to draw to itself a due proportion of blood?

Now, this fluid would be in due proportion if it were so thin and vaporous, that, as soon as it was drawn like dew into every part of the semen, it would everywhere cease to display its own particular character; for so the semen will easily dominate and quickly assimilate it—in fact, will use it as food. It will then, I imagine, draw to itself a second and a third quantum, and thus by feeding it acquires for itself considerable bulk and quantity. In fact, the alterative faculty has now been discovered as well, although about this also has not been written a word. And, thirdly, the shaping faculty will become evident, by virtue of which the semen firstly surrounds itself with a thin membrane like a kind of superficial condensation; this is what was described by Hippocrates in the sixth-day birth, which, according to his statement, fell from the singing-girl and resembled the pellicle of an egg. And following this all the other stages will occur, such as are described by him in his work *On the Child's Nature.* But if each of the parts formed were to remain as small as when it first came into existence, of what use would that be? They have, then, to grow. Now, how will they grow? By becoming extended in all directions and at the same time receiving nourishment. And if you will recall what I previously said about the bladder which the children blew up and rubbed, you will also understand my meaning better as expressed in what I am now about to say. Imagine the heart to be, at the beginning, so small as to differ in no respect from a millet-seed, or, if you will, a bean; and consider how otherwise it is to become large than by being extended in all directions and acquiring nourishment throughout its whole substance, in the way that, as I showed a short while ago, the semen is nourished. But even this was unknown to Erasistratus—the man who sings the artistic skill of Nature! He imagines that animals grow like webs, ropes, sacks, or baskets, each of which has, woven on to its end or margin, other material similar to that of which it was originally composed. But this, most sapient sir, is not growth, but genesis! For a bag, sack, garment, house, ship, or the like is said to be still coming into existence [undergoing genesis] so long as the appropriate form for the sake of which it is being constructed by the artificer is still incomplete. Then, when does it grow? Only when the basket, being complete, with a bottom, a mouth, and a belly, as it were, as well as the intermediate parts, now becomes larger in all these respects. "And how can this happen?" someone will ask. Only by our basket suddenly becoming an animal or a plant; for growth belongs to living things alone. Possibly you imagine that a house grows when it is being built, or a basket when being plated, or a garment when being woven? It is not so, however. Growth belongs to that which has already been completed in respect to its form, whereas the process by which that which is still becoming attains its form is termed not growth but genesis. That which is, grows, while that which is not, becomes.

4 This also was unknown to Erasistratus, whom nothing escaped, if his followers speak in any way truly in maintaining that he was familiar with the Peripatetic philosophers. Now, in so far as he acclaims Nature as being an artist in construction, even I recognize the Peripatetic teachings, but in other respects he does not come near them. For if anyone will make himself acquainted with the writings of Aristotle and Theophrastus, these will appear to him to consist of commentaries on the Nature-lore [physiology] of Hippocrates—according to which the principles of heat, cold, dryness and moisture act upon and are acted upon by one another, the hot principle being the most active, and the cold coming next to it in power; all this was stated in the first place by Hippocrates and secondly by Aristotle. Further, it is at once the Hippocratic and the Aristotelian teaching that the parts which receive that nourishment throughout their whole substance, and that, similarly, processes of mingling and alteration—a transmutation of the nutriment into the proper quality of the thing receiving it; that blood-production also is an alteration, and nutrition as well; that growth results from extension in all directions, combined with nutrition; that alteration is effected mainly by the warm principle, and that therefore digestion, nutrition, and the generation of the various humours, as well as the qualities of the surplus substances, result from the innate heat; all these and many other points besides in regard to the aforesaid faculties, the origin of diseases, and the discovery of remedies, were correctly stated first by Hippocrates of all writers whom we know, and were in the second place correctly expounded by Aristotle. Now, if all these views meet with the approval of the Peripatetics, what can the Erasistrateans possibly mean by claiming that their leader was associated with these philosophers? The fact is, they revere him as a god, and think that everything he says is true. If this be so, then we must suppose the Peripatetics to have strayed very far from the truth, since they approve of none of the ideas of Erasistratus. And, indeed, the disciples of the latter produce his connection with the Peripatetics in order to furnish his Nature-lore with a respectable pedigree.

Now, let us reverse our argument and put it in a different way from that which we have just employed. For if the Peripatetics were correct in their teaching about Nature, there could be nothing more absurd than the contentions of Erasistratus. And, I will leave it to the Erasistrateans themselves to decide; they must either advance the one proposition or the other. According to the former one the Peripatetics had no accurate acquaintance with Nature, and according to the second, Erasistratus. It is my task, then, to point out the opposition between the two doctrines, and theirs to make the choice. . . . But they certainly will not abandon their reverence for Erasistratus. Very well, then; let them stop talking about the Peripatetic philosophers. For among the numerous physiological teachings regarding the genesis and destruction of animals, their health, their diseases, and the methods of treating these, there will not be found one only which is common to Erasistratus and the Peripatetics—namely, the view that Nature does everything for some purpose, and nothing in vain. But even as regards this doctrine their agreement is only verbal; in practice Erasistratus makes havoc of it a thousand times over. For, according to him, the spleen was made for no purpose, as also the omentum; similarly, too, the arteries which are inserted into kidneys—although these are practically the largest of all those that spring from the great artery [aorta]! And to judge by the Erasistratean argument, there must be countless other useless structures; for, if he knows nothing at all about these structures, he has little more anatomical knowledge than a butcher, while, if he is acquainted with them and yet does not state their use, he clearly imagines that they were made for no purpose, like the spleen. Why, however, should I discuss these structures fully, belonging as they do to the treatise *On the Use of Parts,* which I am personally about to complete?

Let us, then, sum up again this same argument, and, having said a few words more in answer to the Erasistrateans, proceed to our next topic. The fact is, these people seem to me to have read none of Aristotle's writings, but to have heard from others how great an authority he was on "Nature," and that those of the Porch follow in the steps of his Nature-lore; apparently they then discovered a single one of the current ideas which is common to Aristotle and Erasistratus, and made up some story of a connection between Erasistratus and these people. That Erasistratus, however, has no share in the Nature-lore of Aristotle is shown by an enumeration of the aforesaid doctrines, which emanated first from Hippocrates, secondly from Aristotle, thirdly from the Stoics (with a single modification, namely, that for them the qualities are bodies). Perhaps, however, they will maintain that it was in the matter of logic that Erasistratus associated himself with the Peripatetic philosophers? Here they show ignorance of the fact that these philosophers never brought forward false or inconclusive arguments, while the Erasistratean books are full of them. So perhaps somebody may already be asking, in some surprise, what possessed Erasistratus that he turned so completely from the doctrines of Hippocrates, and why it is that he takes away the attractive faculty from the biliary passages in the liver—for we have sufficiently discussed the kidneys—alleging [as the cause of bile-secretion] a favourable situation, the narrowness of vessels, and a common space into which the veins from the gateway [of the liver] conduct the unpurified blood, and from which, in the first place, the [biliary] passages take over the bile, and secondly, the [branches] of the vena cava take over the purified blood. For it would not only have done him no harm to have mentioned the idea of attraction, but he would thereby have been able to get rid of countless other disputed questions.

5 At the actual moment, however, the Erasistrateans are engaged in a considerable battle, not only with others but also amongst themselves, and so they cannot explain the passage from the first book of the "General Principles," in which Erasistratus says, "Since there are two kinds of vessels opening at the same place, the one kind extending to the gall-bladder and the other to the vena cava, the result is that, of the nutriment carried up from the alimentary canal, that part which fits both kinds of stomata is received into both kinds of vessels, some being carried into the gall-bladder, and the rest passing over into the vena cava." For it is difficult to say what we are to understand by the words "opening at the same place" which are written at the beginning of this passage. Either they mean there is a junction between the termination of the vein which is on the concave surface of the liver and two other vascular terminations (that of the vessel on the convex surface of the liver and that of the bile-duct), or, if not, then we must suppose that there is, as it were, a common space for all three vessels, which becomes filled from the lower vein and empties itself both into the bile-duct and into the branches of the vena cava. Now, there are many difficulties in both of these explanations, but if I were to state them all, I should find myself inadvertently writing an exposition of the teaching of Erasistratus, instead of carrying out my original undertaking.

There is, however, one difficulty common to both these explanations, namely, that the whole of the blood does not become purified. For it ought to fall into the bile-duct as into a kind of sieve, instead of going (running, in fact, rapidly) past it, into the larger stoma, by virtue of the impulse of anadosis. Are these, then, the only inevitable difficulties in which the argument of Erasistratus becomes involved through his disinclination to make any use of the attractive faculty, or is it that the difficulty is greatest here, and also so obvious that even a child could not avoid seeing it?

6 And if one looks carefully into the matter one will find that even Erasistratus' reasoning on the subject of nutrition, which he takes up in the second book of his "General Principles," fails to escape this same difficulty. For, having conceded one premise to the principle that matter tends to fill a vacuum, as we previously showed, he was only able to draw a conclusion in the case of the veins and their contaminated blood. That is to say, when blood is running away through the stomata of the veins, and is being dispersed, then, since an absolutely empty space cannot result, and the veins cannot collapse (for this was what he overlooked), it was therefore shown to be necessary that the adjoining quantum of fluid should flow in and fill the place of the fluid evacuated. It is in this way that we may suppose the veins to be nourished; they get the benefit of the blood which they contain. But how about the nerves? For they do not also contain blood. One might obviously say that they draw their supply from the veins. But Erasistratus will not have it so. What further contrivance, then, does he suppose? He says that a nerve has within itself veins and arteries, like a rope woven by Nature out of three different strands. By means of this hypothesis he imagined that his theory would escape from the idea of attraction. For if the nerve contain within itself a blood-vessel it will no longer need the adventitious flow of other blood from the real vein lying adjacent; this fictitious vessel, perceptible only in theory, will suffice it for nourishment. But this, again, is succeeded by another similar difficulty. For this small vessel will nourish itself, but it will not be able to nourish this adjacent simple nerve or artery, unless these possess some innate proclivity for attracting nutriment. For how could the nerve, being simple, attract its nourishment, as do the composite veins, by virtue of the tendency of a vacuum to become refilled? For, although according to Erasistratus, it contains within itself a cavity of sorts, this is not occupied with blood, but with psychic pneuma, and we are required to imagine the nutriment introduced, not into this cavity, but into the vessel containing it, whether it needs merely to be nourished, or to grow as well. How, then, are we to imagine it introduced? For this simple vessel [i.e. nerve] is so small—as are also the other two—that if you prick it at any part with the finest needle you will tear the whole three of them at once. Thus there could never be in it a perceptible space entirely empty. And an emptied space which merely existed in theory could not compel the adjacent fluid to come and fill it.

At this point, again, I should like Erasistratus himself to answer regarding this small elementary nerve, whether it is actually one and definitely continuous, or whether it consists of many small bodies, such as those assumed by Epicurus, Leucippus and Democritus. For I see that the Erasistrateans are at variance on this subject. Some of them consider it one and continuous, for otherwise, as they say, he would not have called it simple; and some venture to resolve it into yet other elementary bodies. But if it be one and continuous, then what is evacuated from it in the so-called insensible transpiration of the physicians will leave no empty space in it; otherwise it would not be one body but many, separated by empty spaces. But if it consists of many bodies, then we have "escaped by the back door," as the saying is, to Asclepiades, seeing that we have postulated certain inharmonious elements. Once again, then, we must call Nature "inartistic"; for this necessarily follows the assumption of such elements. For this reason some of the Erasistrateans seem to me to have done very foolishly in reducing the simple vessels to elements such as these. Yet it makes no difference to me, since the theory of both parties regarding nutrition will be shown to be absurd. For in these minute simple vessels constituting the large perceptible nerves, it is impossible, according to the theory of those who would keep the former continuous, that any "refilling of a vacuum" should take place, since no vacuum can occur in a continuum even if anything does run away; for the parts left come together (as is seen in the case of water) and again become one, taking up the whole space of that which previously separated them. Nor will any "refilling" occur if we accept the argument of other Erasistrateans, since none of their elements need it. For this principle only holds of things which are perceptible, and not of those which exist merely in theory; this Erasistratus expressly acknowledges, for he states that it is not a vacuum such as this, interspersed in small portions among the corpuscles, that his various treatises deal with, but a vacuum which is clear, perceptible, complete in itself, large in size, evident, or however else one cares to term it (for, what Erasistratus himself says is, that "there cannot be a perceptible space which is entirely empty"; while I, for my part, being abundantly equipped with terms which are equally elucidatory, at least in relation to the present topic of discussion, have added them as well). Thus it seems to me better that we also should help the Erasistrateans with some contribution, since we are on the subject, and should advise those who reduce the vessel called primary and simply by Erasistratus into other elementary bodies to give up their opinion; for not only do they gain nothing by it, but they are also at variance with Erasistratus in this matter. That they gain nothing by it has been clearly demonstrated; for this hypothesis could not escape the difficulty regarding nutrition.

And it also seems perfectly evident to me that this hypothesis is not in consonance with the view of Erasistratus, when it declares that what he calls simple and primary is composite, and when it destroys the principle of Nature's artistic skill. For, if we do not grant a certain unity of substance to these simple structures as well, and if we arrive eventually at inharmonious and indivisible elements, we shall most assuredly deprive Nature of her artistic skill, as do all the physicians and philosophers who start from this hypothesis. For, according to such a hypothesis, Nature does not precede, but is secondary to the parts of the animal. Now, it is not the province of what comes secondarily, but of what pre-exists, to shape and to construct. Thus we must necessarily suppose that the faculties of Nature, by which she shapes the animal, and makes it grow and receive nourishment, are present from the seed onwards; whereas none of these inharmonious and non-partite corpuscles contains within itself any formative, incremental, nutritive, or, in a word, any artistic power; it is, by hypothesis, unimpressionable and untransformable, whereas, as we have previously shown, none of the processes mentioned takes place without transformation, alteration, and complete intermixture. And, owing to this necessity, those who belong to these sects are unable to follow out the consequences of their supposed elements, and they are all therefore forced to declare Nature devoid of art. It is not from us, however, that the Erasistrateans should have learnt this, but from those very philosophers who lay most stress on a preliminary investigation into the elements of all existing things.

Now, one can hardly be right in supposing that Erasistratus could reach such a pitch of foolishness as to be recognizing the logical consequences of this theory, and that, while assuming Nature to be artistically creative, he would at the same time break up substance into insensible, inharmonious, and untransformable elements. If, however, he will grant that there occurs in the elements a process of alteration and transformation, and that there exists in them unity and continuity, then that simple vessel of his (as he himself names it) will turn out to be single and uncompounded. And the simple vein will receive nourishment from itself, and the nerve and artery from the vein. How, and in what way? For, when we were at this point before, we drew attention to the disagreement among the Erasistrateans, and we showed that the nutrition of these simple vessels was impracticable according to the teachings of both parties, although we did not hesitate to adjudicate in their quarrel and to do Erasistratus the honour of placing him in the better sect. Let out argument, then, be transferred again to the doctrine which assumes this elementary nerve to be a single, simply, and entirely unified structure, and let us consider how it is to be nourished; for what is discovered here will at once be found to be common also to the school of Hippocrates. It seems to me that our enquiry can be most rigorously pursued in subjects who are suffering from illness and have become very emaciated, since in these people all parts of the body are obviously atrophied and thin, and in need of additional substance and feeding-up; for the same reason the ordinary perceptible nerve, regarding which we originally began this discussion, has become thin, and requires nourishment. Now, this contains within itself various parts, namely, a great many of these primary, invisible, minute nerves, a few simple arteries, and similarly also veins. Thus, all its elementary nerves have themselves also obviously become emaciated; for, if they had not, neither would the nerve as a whole; and of course, in such a case, the whole nerve cannot require nourishment without each of these requiring it too. Now, if on the other hand they stand in need of feeding-up, and if on the other the principle of the refilling of a vacuum can give them no help—both by reason of the difficulties previously mentioned and the actual thinness, as I shall show—we must then seek another cause for nutrition. How is it, then, that the tendency of a vacuum to become refilled is unable to afford nourishment to one in such a condition? Because its rule is that only so much of the contiguous matter should succeed as has flowed away. Now this is sufficient for nourishment in the case of those who are in good condition, for, in them, what is presented must be equal to what has flowed away. But in the case of those who are very emaciated and who need a great restoration of nutrition, unless what was presented were many times greater than what has been emptied out, they would never be able to regain their original habit.

It is clear, therefore, that these parts will have to exert a greater amount of attraction, in so far as their requirements are greater. And I fail to understand how Erasistratus does not perceive that here again he is putting the cart before the horse. Because, in the case of the sick, there must be a large amount of presentation in order to feed them up, he argues that the factor of "refilling" must play an equally large part. And how could much presentation take place if it were not preceded by an abundant delivery of nutriment? And if he calls the conveyance of food through the veins delivery, and its assumption by each of these simple and visible nerves and arteries not delivery but distribution, as some people have thought fit to name it, and then ascribes conveyance through the veins to the principle of vacuum refilling alone, let him explain to us the assumption of food by the hypothetical elements. For it has been shown that at least in relation to these there is no question of the refilling of a vacuum being in operation, and especially where the parts are very attenuated. It is worth while listening to what Erasistratus says about these cases in the second book of his "General Principles": "In the ultimate simple [vessels], which are thin and narrow, presentation takes place from the adjacent vessels, the nutriment being attracted through the sides of the vessels and deposited in the empty spaces left by the matter which has been carried away." Now, in this statement firstly I admit and accept the words "through the sides." For, if the simple nerve were actually to take in the food through its mouth, it could not distribute it through its whole substance; for the mouth is dedicated to the psychic pneuma. It can, however, take it in through its sides from the adjacent simple vein. Secondly, I also accept in Erasistratus' statement the expression which precedes "through the sides." What does this say? "The nutriment being attracted through the sides of the vessels." Now I, too, agree that it is attracted, but it has been previously shown that this is not through the tendency of evacuated matter to be replaced.

7 Let us, then, consider together how it is attracted. How else than in the way that iron is attracted by the lodestone, the latter having a faculty attractive of this particular quality [existing in iron]? But if the beginning of anadosis depends on the squeezing action of the stomach, and the whole movement thereafter on the peristalsis and propulsive action of the veins, as well as on the traction exerted by each of the parts which are undergoing nourishment, then we can abandon the principle of replacement of evacuated matter, as not being suitable for a man who assumes Nature to be a skilled artist; thus we shall also have avoided the contradiction of Asclepiades though we cannot refute it: for the disjunctive argument used for the purposes of demonstration is, in reality, disjunctive not of two but of three alternatives, one of the two propositions assumed in constructing our proof must be false; and if as a disjunctive of three alternatives, no conclusion will be arrived at.

8 Now Erasistratus ought not to have been ignorant of this if he had ever had anything to do with the Peripatetics—even in a dream. Nor, similarly, should he have been unacquainted with the genesis of the humours, about which, not having even anything moderately plausible to say, he thinks to deceive us by the excuse that the consideration of such matters is not the least useful. Then, in Heaven's name, is it useful to know how food is digested in the stomach, but unnecessary to know how bile comes into existence in the veins? Are we to pay attention merely to the evacuation of this humour, and not to its genesis? As though it were not far better to prevent its excessive development from the beginning than to give ourselves all the trouble of expelling it! And it is a strange thing to be entirely unaware as to whether its genesis is to be looked on as taking place in the body, or whether it comes from without and is contained in the food. For, if it was right to raise this problem, why should we not make investigations concerning the blood as well—whether it takes its origin in the body, or is distributed through the food as is maintained by those who postulate homoeomeries? Assuredly it would be much more useful to investigate what kinds of food are suited, and what kinds unsuited, to the process of blood-production rather than to enquire into what articles of diet are easily mastered by the activity of the stomach, and what resist and contend with it. For the choice of the latter bears reference merely to digestion, while that of the former is of importance in regard to the generation of useful blood. For it is not equally important whether the aliment be imperfectly chylified in the stomach or whether it fail to be turned into useful blood.

Why is Erasistratus not ashamed to distinguish all the various kinds of digestive failure and all the occasions which give rise to them, whilst in reference to the errors of blood-production he does not utter a single word—nay, not a syllable? Now, there is certainly to be found in the veins both thick and thin blood; in some people it is redder, in others yellower, in some blacker, in others more of the nature of phlegm. And one who realizes that it may smell offensively not in one way only, but in a great many different respects (which cannot be put into words, although perfectly appreciable to the senses), would, I imagine, condemn in no measured terms the carelessness of Erasistratus in omitting a consideration so essential to the practice of our art. Thus it is clear what errors in regard to the subject of dropsies logically follow this carelessness. For, does it not show the most extreme carelessness to suppose that the blood is prevented from going forward into the liver owing to the narrowness of the passages, and that dropsy can never occur in any other way? For, to imagine that dropsy is never caused by the spleen or any other part, but always by induration of the liver is the standpoint of a man whose intelligence is perfectly torpid and who is quite out of touch with things that happen every day. For, not merely once or twice, but frequently, we have observed dropsy produced by chronic haemorrhoids which have been suppressed, or which, through immoderate bleeding, have given the patient a severe chill; similarly, in women, the complete disappearance of the monthly discharge, or an undue evacuation such as is caused by violent bleeding from the womb, often provoke dropsy; and in some of them the so-called female flux ends in this disorder. I leave out of account the dropsy which begins in the flanks or in any other susceptible part; this clearly confutes Erasistratus' assumption, although not so obviously as does that kind of dropsy which is brought about by an excessive chilling of the whole constitution; this, which is the primary reason for the occurrence of dropsy, results from a failure of blood-production, very much like the diarrhoea which follows imperfect digestion of food; certainly in this kind of dropsy neither the liver nor any other viscus becomes indurated.

The learned Erasistratus, however, overlooks—nay, despises—what neither Hippocrates, Diocles, Praxagoras, nor indeed any of the best philosophers, whether Plato, Aristotle, or Theophrastus; he passes by whole functions as though it were but a trifling and casual department of medicine which he was neglecting, without deigning to argue whether or not these authorities are right in saying that the bodily part of all animals are governed by the Warm, the Cold, the Dry and the Moist, the one pair being active the other passive, and that among these the Warm has most power in connection with all functions, but especially with the genesis of the humours. Now, one cannot be blamed for not agreeing with all these great men, nor for imagining that one knows more than they; but not to consider such distinguished teaching worthy either of contradiction or even mention shows an extraordinary arrogance. Now, Erasistratus is thoroughly small-minded and petty to the last degree in all his disputations—when, for instance, in his treatise *On Digestion,* he argues jealously with those who consider that this is a process of putrefaction of the food; and, in his work *On Anadosis,* with those who think that the anadosis of blood through the veins results from the contiguity of the arteries; also, in his work *On Respiration,* with those who maintain that the air is forced along by contraction. Nay, he did not hesitate to contradict those who maintain that the urine passes into the bladder in a vaporous state, as also those who say that imbibed fluids are carried into the lung. Thus he delights to choose always the most valueless doctrines, and to spend his time more and more in contradicting these; whereas on the subject of the origin of blood (which is in no way less important than the chylification of food in the stomach) he did not deign to dispute with any of the ancients, nor did he himself venture to bring forward any other opinion, despite the fact that at the beginning of his treatise on

"General Principles" he undertook to say how all the various natural functions take place, and through what parts of the animal!

Now, is it possible that, when the faculty which naturally digests food is weak, the animal's digestion fails, whereas the faculty which turns the digested food into blood cannot suffer any kind of impairment? Are we to suppose this latter faculty alone to be as tough as steel and unaffected by circumstances? Or is it that weakness of this faculty will result in something else than dropsy? The fact, therefore, that Erasistratus, in regard to other matters, did not hesitate to attack even the most trivial views, whilst in this he neither dared to contradict his predecessors nor to advance any new view of his own, proves plainly that he recognized the fallacy of his own way of thinking. For what could a man possibly say about blood who had no use for innate heat? What could he say about yellow or black bile, or phlegm? Well, of course, he might say that the bile could come directly from without, mingled with the food! Thus Erasistratus practically says so in the following words: "It is of no value in practical medicine to find out whether fluid of this kind arises from the elaboration of food in the stomach-region, or whether it reaches the body because it is mixed with the food taken in from outside." But my very good Sir, you most certainly maintain also that this humour has to be evacuated from the animal, and that it causes great pain if it be not evacuated. How, then, if you suppose that no good comes from the bile, do you venture to say that an investigation into its origin is of no value in medicine? Well, let us suppose that it is contained in the food, and not specifically secreted in the liver (for you hold these two things possible). In this case, it will certainly make a considerable difference whether the ingested food contains a minimum or a maximum of bile; for the one kind is harmless, whereas that containing a large quantity of bile, owing to the fact that it cannot be properly purified in the liver, will result in the various affections—particularly jaundice—which Erasistratus himself states to occur where there is much bile. Surely, then, it is most essential for the physician to know in the first place, that the bile is contained in the food itself from outside, and, secondly, that for example, beet contains a great deal of bile, and bread very little, while olive oil contains most, and wine least of all, and all the other articles of diet different quantities. Would it not be absurd for any one to choose voluntarily those articles which contain more bile, rather than those containing less? What, however, if the bile is not contained in the food, but comes into existence in the animal's body? Will it not also be useful to know what state of the body is followed by a greater, and what by a smaller occurrence of bile? For obviously it is in our power to alter and transmute morbid states of the body—in fact, to give them a turn for the better. But if we did not know in what respect they were morbid or in what way they diverged from the normal, how should we be able to ameliorate them?

Therefore it is not useless in treatment, as Erasistratus says, to know the actual truth about the genesis of bile. Certainly it is not impossible, or even difficult to discover that the reason why honey produces yellow bile is not that it contains a large quantity of this within itself, but because it [the honey] undergoes change, becoming altered and transmuted into bile. For it would be better to the taste if it contained bile from the outset, and it would produce an equal quantity of bile in every person who took it. The facts, however, are not so. For in those who are in the prime of life, especially if they are warm by nature and are leading a life of toil, the honey changes entirely into yellow bile. Old people, however, it suits well enough, inasmuch as the alteration which it undergoes is not into bile, but into blood. Erasistratus, however, in addition to knowing nothing about this, shows no intelligence even in the division of his argument; he says that it is of no practical importance to investigate whether the bile is contained in the food from the beginning or comes into existence as a result of gastric digestion. He ought surely to have added something about its genesis in liver and veins, seeing that the old physicians and philosophers declare that it along with the blood is generated in these organs.

But it is inevitable that people who, from the very outset, go astray, and wander from the right road, should talk such nonsense, and should, over and above this, neglect to search for the factors of most practical importance in medicine. Having come to the point in the argument, I should like to ask those who declare that Erasistratus was very familiar with the Peripatetics, whether they know what Aristotle stated and demonstrated with regard to our bodies being compounded out of the Warm, the Cold, the Dry and the Moist, and how he says that among these the Warm is the most active, and that those animals which are by nature warmest have abundance of blood, whilst those that are colder are entirely lacking in blood, and consequently in winter lie idle and motionless, lurking in holes like corpses. Further, the question of the colour of the blood has been dealt with not only by Aristotle but also by Plato. Now I, for my part, as I have already said, did not set before myself the task of stating what has been so well demonstrated by the Ancients, since I cannot surpass these men either in my views or in my method of giving them expression. Doctrines, however, which they either stated without demonstration, as being self-evident (since they never suspected that there could be sophists so degraded as to contemn the truth in these matters), or else which they actually omitted to mention at all—these I propose to discover and prove.

Now in reference to the genesis of the humours, I do not know that any one could add anything wiser than what has been said by Hippocrates, Aristotle, Praxagoras, Philotimus and many others among the Ancients. These men demonstrated that when the nutriment becomes altered in the veins by the innate heat, blood is produced when it is in moderation, and the other humours when it is not in proper proportion. And all the observed facts agree with this argument. Thus, those articles of food, which are by nature warmer are more productive of bile, while those which are colder produce more phlegm. Similarly of the periods of life, those which are naturally warmer tend more to bile, and the colder more to phlegm. Of occupations also, localities and seasons, and, above all, of natures themselves, the colder are more phlegmatic, and the warmer more bilious. Also cold diseases result from phlegm and warmer ones from yellow bile. There is not a single thing to be found which does not bear witness to the truth of this account. How could it be otherwise? For, seeing that every part functions in its own special way because of the manner in which the four qualities are compounded, it is absolutely necessary that the function [activity] should be either completely destroyed, or, at least hampered, by any damage to the qualities, and that thus the animal should fall ill, either as a whole, or in certain of its parts. Also the diseases which are primary and most generic are four in number, and differ from each other in warmth, cold, dryness and moisture. Now, Erasistratus himself confesses this, albeit unintentionally; for when he says that the digestion of food becomes worse in fever, not because the innate heat has ceased to be in due proportion, as people previously supposed, but because the stomach, with its activity impaired, cannot contract and triturate as before—then, I say, one may justly ask him what it is that has impaired the activity of the stomach.

Thus, for example, when a bubo develops following an accidental wound gastric digestion does not become impaired until the patient has become fevered; neither the bubo nor the sore of itself impedes in any way or damages the activity of the stomach. But if fever occurs, the digestion at once deteriorates, and we are also right in saying that the activity of the stomach at once becomes impaired. We must add, however, by what it has been impaired. For the wound was not capable of impairing it, nor yet the bubo, for, if they had been, then they would have caused this damage before the fever as well. If it was not these that caused it, then it was the excess of heat (for these two symptoms occurred besides the bubo—an alteration in the arterial and cardiac movements and an excessive development of natural heat). Now the alteration of these movements will not merely not impair the function of the stomach in any way: it will actually prove an additional help among those animals in which, according to Erasistratus, the pneuma, which is propelled through the arteries and into the alimentary canal, is of great service in digestion; there is only left, then, the disproportionate heat to account for the damage to the gastric activity. For the pneuma is driven in more vigorously and continuously, and in greater quantity now than before; thus in this case, the animal whose digestion is promoted by pneuma will digest more, whereas the remaining factor—abnormal heat—will give them indigestion. For to say, on the one hand, that the pneuma has a certain property by virtue of which it promotes digestion, and then to say that this property disappears in cases of fever, is simply to admit the absurdity. For when they are again asked what it is that has altered the pneuma, they will only be able to reply, "the abnormal heat," and particularly if it be the pneuma in the food canal which is in question (since this does not come in any way near the bubo).

Yet why do I mention those animals in which the property of the pneuma plays an important part, when it is possible to base one's argument upon human beings, in whom it is either of no importance at all, or acts quite faintly and feebly? But Erasistratus himself agrees that human beings digest badly in fevers, adding as the cause that the activity of the stomach has been impaired. He cannot, however, advance any other cause of this impairment than abnormal heat. But if it is not by accident that the abnormal heat impairs this activity, but by virtue of its own essence and power, then this abnormal heat must belong to the primary diseases. But, indeed, if disproportion of heat belongs to the primary diseases, it cannot but be that a proportionate blending [eucrasia] of the qualities produces the normal activity. For a disproportionate blend [dyscrasia] can only become a cause of the primary diseases through derangement of the eucrasia. That is to say, it is because the [normal] activities arise from the eucrasia that the primary impairments of these activities arise from the derangement. I think, then, it has been proved to the satisfaction of those who are capable of seeing logical consequences, that, even according to Erasistratus' own argument, the cause of the normal functions is eucrasia of the Warm. Now, this being so, there is nothing further to prevent us from saying that, in the case of each function, eucrasia is followed by the more, and dyscrasia by the less favourable alternative. And, therefore, if this be the case, we must suppose blood to be the outcome of proportionate, and yellow bile of disproportionate heat. So we naturally find yellow bile appearing in greatest quantity in ourselves at the warm periods of life, in warm countries, at warm seasons of the year, and when we are in a warm condition; similarly in people of warm temperaments, and in connection with warm occupations, modes of life, or diseases. And to be in doubt as to whether this humour has the genesis in the human body or is contained in the food is what you would expect from one who has—I will not say failed to see that, when those who are perfectly healthy have, under the compulsion of circumstances, to fast contrary to custom, their mouths become bitter and their urine bile-coloured, while they suffer from gnawing pains in the stomach—but has, as it were, just made a sudden entrance into the world, and is not yet familiar with the phenomena which occur there. Who, in fact, does not know that anything which is overcooked grows at first salty and afterwards bitter? And if you will boil honey itself, far the sweetest of things, you can demonstrate that even this becomes quite bitter. For what may occur as a result of boiling in the case of other articles which are not warm by nature, exists naturally in honey; for this reason it does not become sweeter on being boiled, since exactly the same quantity of heat as is needed for the production of sweetness exists from beforehand in the honey. Therefore the external heat, which would be useful for insufficiently warm substances, becomes in the honey a source of damage, in fact an excess; and it is for this reason that honey, when boiled, can be demonstrated to become bitter sooner than the others.

For the same reason it is easily transmuted into bile in those people who are naturally warm, or in their prime, since warm when associated with warm becomes readily changed into a disproportionate combination and turns into bile sooner than into blood. Thus we need a cold temperament and a cold period of life if we would have honey brought to the nature of blood. Therefore Hippocrates not improperly advised those who were naturally bilious not to take honey, since they were obviously of too warm a temperament. So also, not only Hippocrates, but all physicians say that honey is bad in bilious diseases but good in old age; some of them having discovered this through the indications afforded by its nature, and others simply through experiment, for the Empiricist physicians too have made precisely the same observation, namely, that honey is good for an old man and not for a young one, that it is harmful for those who are naturally bilious, and serviceable for those who are phlegmatic. In a word, in bodies which are warm either through nature, disease, time of life, season of the year, locality, or occupation, honey is productive of bile, whereas in opposite circumstances it produces blood. But surely it is impossible that the same article of diet can produce in certain persons bile and in others blood, and did not produce it by undergoing change in the animal body, then they would produce it similarly in all bodies; the food which was bitter to the taste would, I take it, be productive of bile, while that which tasted good and sweet would not generate even the smallest quantity of bile. Moreover, not only honey but all other sweet substances are readily converted into bile in the aforesaid bodies which are warm for any of the reasons mentioned. Well, I have somehow or other been led into this discussion,—not in accordance with my plan, but compelled by the course of the argument. This subject has been treated at great length by Aristotle and Praxagoras, who have correctly expounded the view of Hippocrates and Plato.

9 For this reason the things that we have said are not to be looked upon as proofs but rather as indications of the dullness of those who think differently, and who do not even recognise what is agreed on by everyone and is a matter of daily observation. As for the scientific proofs of all this, they are to be drawn from these principles of which I have already spoken—namely, that bodies act upon and are acted upon by each other in virtue of the Warm, Cold, Moist and Dry. And if one is speaking of any activity, whether it be exercised by vein, liver, arteries, heart, alimentary canal, or any part, one will be inevitably compelled to acknowledge that this activity depends on the way in which the four qualities are blended. Thus I should like to ask the Erasistrateans why it is that the stomach contracts upon the food, and why the veins generate blood. There is no use in recognizing the mere fact of contraction, without also knowing the cause; if we know this, we shall also be able to rectify the failures of function. "This is no concern of ours," they say; "we do not occupy ourselves with such causes as these; they are outside the sphere of the practitioner, and belong to that of the scientific investigator." Are you, then, going to oppose those who maintain that the cause of the function of every organ is a natural eucrasia, that the dyscrasia is itself known as a disease, and that it is certainly by this that the activity becomes impaired? Or, on the other hand, will you be convinced by the proofs which the ancient writers furnished? Or will you take a midway course between these two, neither perforce accepting these arguments as true nor contradicting them as false, but suddenly becoming sceptics—Pyrrhonists, in fact? But if you do this you will have to shelter yourselves behind the Empiricist teaching. For how are you going to be successful in treatment, if you do not understand the real essence of each disease? Why, then, did you not call yourselves Empiricists from the beginning? Why do you confuse us by announcing that you are investigating natural activities with a view to treatment? If the stomach is, in a particular case, unable to exercise its peristaltic and grinding functions, how are we going to bring it back to the normal if we do not know the cause of its disability? What I say is that we must cool the over-heated stomach and warm the chilled one; so also we must moisten the one which has become dried up, and conversely; so, too, in combinations of these conditions; if the stomach becomes at the same time warmer and drier than normally, the first principle treatment is at once to chill and moisten it; and if it become colder and moister, it must be warmed and dried; so also in other cases. But how on earth are the followers of Erasistratus going to act, confessing as they do that they make no sort of investigation into the cause of disease? For the fruit of the enquiry into activities is that by knowing the causes of the dycrasiae one may bring them back to the normal, since it is of no use for the purposes of treatment merely to know what the activity of each organ is.

Now, it seems to me that Erasistratus is unaware of this fact also, that the actual disease is that condition of the body which, not accidentally, but primarily and of itself, impairs the normal function. How, then, is he going to diagnose or cure diseases if he is entirely ignorant of what they are, and of what kind and number? As regards the stomach, certainly, Erasistratus held that one should at least investigate how it digests the food. But why was not investigation also made as to the primary originative cause of this? And, as regards the veins and the blood, he omitted even to ask the question "how?" Yet neither Hippocrates nor any of the other physicians or philosophers whom I mentioned a short while ago thought it right to omit this; they say that when the heat which exists naturally in every animal is well blended and moderately moist it generates blood; for this reason they also say that the blood is a virtually warm and moist humour, and similarly also that yellow bile is warm and dry, even though for the most part it appears moist. (For in them the apparently dry would seem to differ from the virtually dry.) Who does not know that brine and sea-water preserve meat and keep it uncorrupted, while all other water—the drinkable kind—readily spoils and rots it? And who does not know that when yellow bile is contained in large quantity in the stomach, we are troubled with an unquenchable thirst, and that when we vomit this up, we at once become much freer from thirst than if we had drunk very large quantities of fluid? Therefore this humour has been very properly termed warm, and also virtually dry. And, similarly, phlegm has been called cold and moist; for about this clear proofs have been given by Hippocrates and the other Ancients. Prodicus also, when in his book *On the Nature of Man* he gives the name "phlegm" to that element in the humours which has been burned or, as it were, over-roasted, while using a different terminology, still keeps to the fact just as the others do; this man's innovations in nomenclature have also been amply done justice to by Plato.

Thus, the white-coloured substance which everyone else calls phlegm, and which Prodicus calls blenna [mucus], is the well-known cold, moist humour which collects mostly in old people and in those who have been chilled in some way, and not even a lunatic could say that this was anything else than cold and moist. If, then, there is a warm and moist humour, and another which is warm and dry, and yet another which is moist and cold, is there none which is virtually cold and dry? Is the fourth combination of temperaments, which exists in all other things, non-existent in the humours alone? No; the black bile is such a humour. This, according to intelligent physicians and philosophers, tends to be in excess, as regards seasons, mainly in the fall of the year, and, as regards ages, mainly after the prime of life. And, similarly, also they say that there are cold and dry modes of life, regions, constitutions, and diseases. Nature, they suppose, is not defective in this single combination; like the three other combinations, it extends everywhere. At this point, also, I would gladly have been able to ask Erasistratus whether his "artistic" Nature has not constructed any organ for clearing away a humour such as this. For whilst there are two organs for the excretion of urine, and another of considerable size for that of yellow bile, does the humour which is more pernicious than these wander about persistently in the veins mingled with the blood? Yet Hippocrates says, "Dysentery is a fatal condition if it proceeds from black bile"; while that proceeding from yellow bile is by no means deadly, and most people recover from it; this proves how much more pernicious and acrid in its potentialities is black than yellow bile. Has Erasistratus, then, not read the book, *On the Nature of Man,* any more than the rest of Hippocrates' writings, that he so carelessly passes over the consideration of the humours? Or, does he know it, and yet voluntarily neglect one of the finest studies in medicine? Thus he ought not to have said anything about the spleen, nor have stultified himself by holding that an artistic Nature would have prepared so large an organ for no purpose.

As a matter of fact, not a matter of fact, not only Hippocrates and Plato—who are no less authorities on Nature than is Erasistratus—say that this viscus also is one of those which cleanse the blood, but there are thousands of the ancient physicians and philosophers as well who are in agreement with them. Now, all of these the high and mighty Erasistrateans affected to despise, and he neither contradicted them nor even so much as mentioned their opinion. Hippocrates, indeed, says that the spleen wastes in those people in whom the body is in good condition, and all those physicians also who base themselves on experience agree with this. Again, in those cases in which the spleen is large and is increasing from internal suppuration, it destroys the body and fills it with evil humours; this again is agreed on, not only by Hippocrates, but also by Plato and many others, including the Empiric physicians. And the jaundice which occurs when the spleen is out of order is darker in colour, and the cicatrices of ulcers are dark. For, generally speaking, when the spleen is drawing the atrabiliary humour into itself to a less degree than is proper, the blood is unpurified, and the whole body takes on a bad colour. And when does it draw this in to a less degree than proper? Obviously, when it [the spleen] is in a bad condition. Thus, just as the kidneys, whose function it is to attract the urine, do this badly when they are out of order, so also the spleen, which has in itself a native power of attracting an atrabiliary quality, if it ever happens to be weak, must necessarily exercise this attraction badly, with the result that the blood becomes thicker and darker. Now all these points, affording as they do the greatest help in the diagnosis and in the cure of disease were entirely passed over by Erasistratus, and he pretended to despise these great men—he who does not despise ordinary people, but always jealously attacks the most absurd doctrines. Hence, it was clearly because he had nothing to say against the statements made by the Ancients regarding the function and utility of the spleen, and also because he could discover nothing new himself, that he ended by saying nothing at all.

I, however, for my part, have demonstrated, firstly from the causes by which everything throughout nature is governed (by the causes I mean the Warm, Cold, Dry and Moist) and secondly, from obvious bodily phenomena, that there must needs be a cold and dry humour. And having in the next place drawn attention to the fact that this humour is black bile [atrabiliary] and that the viscus which clears it away is the spleen—having pointed this out by help of as few as possible of the proofs given by ancient writers, I shall now proceed to what remains of the subject in hand. What else, then, remains but to explain clearly what it is that happens in the generation of the humours, according to the belief and demonstration of the Ancients? This will be more clearly understood from a comparison. Imagine, then, some new wine which has been not long ago pressed from the grape, and which is fermenting and undergoing alteration through the agency of its contained heat. Imagine next two residual substances produced during this process of alteration, the one tending to be light and air-like and the other to be heavy and more of the nature of earth; of these the one, as I understand, they call the flower and the other the lees. Now you may correctly compare yellow bile to the first of these, and black bile to the latter, although these humours have not the same appearance when the animal is in normal health as that which they often show when it is not so; for then the yellow bile becomes vitelline, being so termed because it becomes like the yolk of an egg, both in colour and density; and again, even the black bile itself becomes much more malignant than when it is in its normal condition, but no particular name has been given to [such a condition of] the humour, except that some people have called it corrosive or acetose, because it also becomes sharp like vinegar and corrodes the animal's body—as also the earth, if it be poured out upon it—and it produces a kind of fermentation and seething, accompanied by bubbles—an abnormal putrefaction having become added to the natural condition of the black humour.

It seems to me also that most of the ancient physicians give the name black humour and not black bile to the normal portion of this humour, which is discharged from the bowel and which also frequently rises to the top [of the stomach-contents]; and they call black bile that part which, through a kind of combustion and putrefaction, has had its quality changed to acid. There is no need, however, to dispute about names, but we must realise the facts, which are as follow:—In the genesis of blood, everything in the nutriment which belongs naturally to the thick and earth-like part of the food, and which does not take on well the alteration produced by the innate heat—all this the spleen draws into itself. On the other hand, that part of the nutriment which is roasted, so to speak, or burnt (this will be the warmest and sweetest part of it, like honey and fat), becomes yellow bile, and is cleared away through the so-called biliary vessels; now, this is thin, moist, and fluid, not like what it is when, having been roasted to an excessive degree, it becomes yellow, fiery, and thick, like the yolk of eggs; for this latter is already abnormal, while the previously mentioned state is natural.

Similarly with the black humour: that which does not yet produce, as I say, this seething and fermentation on the ground, is natural, while that which has taken over this character and faculty is unnatural; it has assumed an acridity owing to the combustion caused by abnormal heart, and has practically become transformed into ashes. In somewhat the same way burned lees differ from unburned. The former is a warm substance, able to burn, dissolve, and destroy the flesh. The other kind, which has not yet undergone combustion, one may find the physicians employing for the same purposes that one uses the so-called potter's earth and other substances which have naturally a combined drying and chilling action. Now the vitelline bile also may take on the appearance of this combusted black bile, if ever it chance to be roasted, so to say, by fiery heat. And all the other forms of bile are produced, some from the blending of those mentioned, others being, as it were, transition-stages in the genesis of these or in their conversion into one another. And they differ in that those first mentioned are unmixed and unique, while the latter forms are diluted with various kinds of serum. And all the serums in the humours are waste substances, and the animal body needs to be purified from them.

There is, however, a natural use for the humours first mentioned, both thick and thin; the blood is purified both by the spleen and by the bladder beside the liver, and a part of each of the two humours is put away, of such quantity and quality that, if it were carried all over the body, it would do a certain amount of harm. For that which is decidedly thick and earthy in nature, and has entirely escaped alteration in the liver, is drawn by the spleen into itself; the other part which is only moderately thick, after being elaborated [in the liver], is carried all over the body. For the blood in many parts of the body has need of a certain amount of thickening, as also, I take it, of the fibres which it contains. And the use of these has been discussed by Plato, and it will also be discussed by me in such of my treatises as may deal with the use of parts. And the blood also needs, not least, the yellow humour, which has as yet not reached the extreme stage of combustion; in the treatises mentioned it will be pointed out what purpose is subserved by this.

Now Nature has made no organ for clearing away phlegm, this being cold and moist, and, as it were, half-digested nutriment; such a substance, therefore, does not need to be evacuated, but remains in the body and undergoes alteration there. And perhaps one cannot properly give the name of phlegm to the surplus-substance which runs down from the brain, but one should call it mucus [blenna] or coryza—as, in fact, it is actually termed; in any case it will be pointed out, in the treatise *On the Use of Parts,* how Nature has provided for the evacuation of this substance. Further, the device provided by Nature which ensures that the phlegm which forms in the stomach and intestines may be evacuated in the most rapid and effective way possible—this also will be described in that commentary. As to that portion of the phlegm which is carried in the veins, seeing that this is of service to the animal, it requires no evacuation. Here too, then, we must pay attention and recognise that, just as in the case of each of the two kinds of bile, there is one part which is useful to the animal and in accordance with its nature, while the other part is useless and contrary to nature, so also is it with the phlegm; such of it as is sweet is useful to the animal and according to nature, while, as to such of it as has become bitter or salty, that part which is bitter is completely undigested, while that part which is salty has undergone putrefaction. And the term "complete indigestion" refers of course to the second digestion—that which takes place in the veins; it is not a failure of the first digestion—that in the alimentary canal—for it would not have become a humour at the outset if it had escaped this digestion also.

It seems to me that I have made enough reference to what has been said regarding the genesis and destruction of humours by Hippocrates, Plato, Aristotle, Praxagoras, and Diocles, and many others among the Ancients; I did not deem it right to transport the whole of their final pronouncements into this treatise. I have said only so much regarding each of the humours as will stir up the reader, unless he be absolutely inept, to make himself familiar with the writings of the Ancients, and will help him to gain more easy access to them. In another treatise I have written on the humours according to Praxagoras, to Praxagoras, son of authority Nicarchus; although this authority makes as many as ten humours, not including the blood (the blood itself being an eleventh), this is not a departure from the teaching of Hippocrates; for Praxagoras divides into species and varieties the humours which Hippocrates first mentioned, with the demonstration proper to each. Those, then, are to be praised who explain the points which have been duly mentioned, as also those who add what has been left out; for it is not possible for the same man to make both a beginning and an end. Those, on the other hand, deserve censure who are so impatient that they will not wait to learn any of the things which have been duly mentioned, as do also those who are so ambitious that, in their lust after novel doctrines, they are always attempting some fraudulent sophistry, either purposefully neglecting certain subjects, as Erasistratus does in the case of the humours, or unscrupulously attacking other people, as does this same writer, as well as many of the more recent authorities. But let this discussion come to an end here, and I shall add in the third book all that remains.

BOOK III

1 It has been made clear in the preceding discussion that nutrition occurs by an alteration or assimilation of that which nourishes to that which receives nourishment, and that there exists in every part of the animal a faculty which in view of its activity we call, in general terms, alterative, or, more specifically, assimilative and nutritive. It was also shown that a sufficient supply of the matter which the part being nourished makes into nutriment for itself is ensured by virtue of another faculty which naturally attracts its proper juice [humour], that that juice is proper to each part which is adapted for assimilation, and that the faculty which attracts the juice is called, by reason of its activity, attractive or epispastic. It has also been shown that assimilation is preceded by adhesion, and this, again, by presentation, the latter stage being, as one might say, the end or goal of the activity corresponding to the attractive faculty. For the actual bringing up of nutriment from the veins into each of the parts takes place through the activation of the attractive faculty, whilst to have been finally brought up and presented to the part is the actual end for which we desired such an activity; it is attracted in order that it may be presented. After this, considerable time is needed for the nutrition of the animal; whilst a thing may be even rapidly attracted, on the other hand to become adherent, altered, and entirely assimilated to the part which is being nourished and to become a part of it, cannot take place suddenly, but requires a considerable amount of time.

But if the nutritive juice, so presented, does not remain in the part, but withdraws to another one, and keeps flowing away, and constantly changing and shifting its position, neither adhesion nor complete assimilation will take place in front of them. Here too, then, the [animal's] nature has need of some other faculty for ensuring a prolonged stay of the presented juice at the part, and this not a faculty which comes in from somewhere outside but one which is resident in the part which is to be nourished. This faculty, again, in view of its activity our predecessors were obliged to call retentive. Thus our argument has clearly shown the necessity for the genesis of such a faculty, and whoever has an appreciation of logical sequence must be firmly persuaded from what we have said that, if it be laid down and proved by previous demonstration that Nature is artistic and solicitous for the animal's welfare, it necessarily follows that she must also possess a faculty of this kind.

2 Since, however, it is not our habit to employ this kind of demonstration alone, but to add thereto cogent and compelling proofs drawn from obvious facts, we will also proceed to the latter kind in the present instance: we will demonstrate that in certain parts of the body the retentive faculty is so obvious that its operation can be actually recognised by the senses, whilst in other parts it is less obvious to the senses, but is capable even here of being detected by the argument. Let us begin our exposition, then, by first dealing systematically for a while with certain definite parts of the body, in reference to which we may accurately test and enquire what sort of thing the retentive faculty is. Now, could one begin the enquiry in any better way than with the largest and hollowest organs? Personally I do not think one could. It is to be expected that in these, owing to their size, the activities will show quite clearly, whereas with respect to the smaller organs, even if they possess a strong faculty of this kind, its activation will not at once be recognisable to sense.

Now those parts of the animal which are especially hollow and large are the stomach and the organ which is called the womb or uterus. What prevents us, then, from taking up these first and considering their activities, conducting the enquiry on our own persons in regard to those activities which are obvious without dissection, and, in the case of those which are more obscure, dissecting animals which are near to man; not that even animals unlike him will not show, in a general way, the faculty in question, but because in this manner we may find out at once what is common to all and what is peculiar to ourselves, and so may become more resourceful in the diagnosis and treatment of disease. Now it is impossible to speak of both organs at once, so we shall deal with each in turn, beginning with the one which is capable of demonstrating the retentive faculty most plainly. For the stomach retains the food until it has quite digested it, and the uterus retains the embryo until it brings it to completion, but the time taken for the completion of the embryo is many times more than that for the digestion of food.

3 We may expect, then, to detect the retentive faculty in the uterus more clearly in proportion to the longer duration of its activity as compare with that of the stomach. For, as we know, it takes nine months in most women for the foetus to attain maturity in the womb, this organ having its neck quite closed, and entirely surrounding the embryo together with the chlorion. Further, it is the utility of the function which determines the closure of the os and the stay of the foetus in the uterus. For it is not casually nor without reason that Nature has made the uterus capable of contracting upon, and of retaining the embryo, but in order that the latter may arrive at a proper size. When, therefore, the object for which the uterus brought its retentive faculty into play has been fulfilled, it then stops this faculty and brings it back to a state of rest, and employs instead of it another faculty hitherto quiescent—the propulsive faculty. In this case again the quiescent and active states are both determined by utility; when this calls, there is activity; when it does not, there is rest. Here, then, once more, we must observe well the Art [artistic tendency] of Nature—how she has not merely placed in each organ the capabilities of useful activities, but has also fore-ordained the times both of rest and movement.

For everything connected with the pregnancy proceeds properly, the eliminative faculty remains quiescent as though it did not exist, but if anything goes wrong in connection either with the chlorion or any of the other membranes or with the foetus itself, and its completion is entirely despaired of, then the uterus no longer awaits the nine-months period, but the retentive faculty forthwith ceases and allows the heretofore inoperative faculty to come into action. Now it is that something is done—in fact, useful work effected—by the eliminative or propulsive faculty (for so it, too, has been called, receiving, like the rest, its names from the corresponding activities). Further, our theory can, I think demonstrate both together; for seeing that they succeed each other, and that the one keeps giving place to the other according as utility demands, it seems not unreasonable to accept a common demonstration also for both. Thus it is the work of the retentive faculty to make the uterus contract upon the foetus at every point, so that, naturally enough, when the midwives palpate it, the os is found to be closed, whilst the pregnant women themselves, during the first days—

and particularly on that on which conception takes place—experience a sensation as if the uterus were moving and contracting upon itself.

Now, if both of these things occur—if the os closes apart from inflammation or any other disease, and if this is accompanied by a feeling of movement in the uterus—then the women believe that they have received the semen which comes from the male, and that they are retaining it. Now we are not inventing this for ourselves: one may say the statement is based on prolonged experience of those who occupy themselves with such matters. Thus Herophilus does not hesitate to state in his writings that up to the time of labour the os uteri will not admit so much as the tip of a probe, that it no longer opens to the slightest degree if pregnancy has begun—that, in fact, it dilates more widely at the times of the menstrual flow. With him are in agreement all the others who have applied themselves to this subject; and particularly Hippocrates, who was the first of all physicians and philosophers to declare that the os uteri closes during pregnancy and inflammation, albeit in pregnancy it does not depart from its own nature, whilst in inflammation it becomes hard. In the case of the opposite (the eliminative) faculty, the os opens, whilst the whole fundus approaches as near as possible to the os, expelling the embryo as it does so; and along with the fundus the contiguous parts—which form as it were a girdle round the whole organ—cooperate in the work; they squeeze upon the embryo and propel it bodily outwards. And, in many women who exercise such a faculty immoderately, violent cause forcible prolapse of the whole womb; here almost the same thing happens as frequently occurs in wresting—bouts and struggles, when in our eagerness to overturn and throw others we are ourselves upset along with them; for similarly when the uterus is forcing the embryo forward it sometimes becomes entirely prolapsed, and particularly when the ligaments connecting it with the spine happen to be naturally lax.

A wonderful device of Nature's also is this—that, when the foetus is alive, the os uteri is closed with perfect accuracy, but if it dies, the os at once opens up to the extent which is necessary for the foetus to make its exit. The midwife, however, does not make the parturient women get up at once and sit down on the [obstetric] chair, but she begins by palpating the os as it gradually dilates, and the first thing she says is that it has dilated "enough to admit the little finger," then that "it is bigger now," and as we make enquiries from time to time, she answers that the size of the dilation is increasing. And when it is sufficient to allow of the transit of the foetus, she then makes the patient get up from her bed and sit on the chair, and bids her make every effort to expel the child. Now, this additional work which the patient does of herself is no longer the work of the uterus but of the epigastric muscles, which also help us in defaecation and micturition.

4 Thus the two faculties are clearly to be seen in the case of the uterus; in the case of the stomach they appear as follows: firstly in the condition of gurgling, which physicians are persuaded, and with reason, to be a symptom of weakness of the stomach; for sometimes when the very smallest quantity food has been ingested this does not occur, owing to the fact that the stomach is contracting accurately upon the food and constricting it at every point; sometimes when the stomach is full the gurglings yet make themselves heard as though it were empty. For if it be in a natural condition, employing its contractile faculty in the ordinary way, then, even if its contents be very small, it grasps the whole of them and does not leave any empty space. When it is weak, however, being unable to lay hold of its contents accurately, it produces a certain amount of vacant space, and amount of vacant space, and allows the liquid contents to flow about in different directions in accordance with its changes of shape, and so to produce gurglings. Thus those who are troubled with this symptom expect, with good reason, that they will also be unable to digest adequately; proper digestion cannot take place in a weak stomach. In such people also, the mass of food may be plainly seen to remain an abnormally long time in the stomach, as would be natural if their digestion were slow.

Indeed, the chief way in which these people will surprise one is in the length of time that not food alone but even fluids will remain in their stomachs. Now, the actual cause of this is not, as one would imagine, that the lower outlet of the stomach, being fairly narrow, will allow nothing to pass before being reduced to a fine state of division. There are a great many people who frequently swallow large quantities of big fruit-stones; one person who was holding a gold ring in his mouth, inadvertently swallowed it; another swallowed a coin, and various people have swallowed various hard and indigestible objects; yet all these people easily passed by the bowel what they had swallowed, without there being any subsequent symptoms. Now surely if narrowness of the gastric outlet were the cause of untriturated food remaining for an abnormally long time, none of these articles I have mentioned would ever have escaped. Furthermore, the fact that it is liquids which remain longest in these people's stomachs is sufficient to put the idea of narrowness of the outlet out of court. For, supposing a rapid descent were dependent upon emulsification, then soups, milk, and barley—emulsion would at once pass along in every case. But as a matter of fact this is not so. For in people who are extremely asthenic it is just these fluids which remain undigested, which accumulate and produce gurglings, and which oppress and overload the stomach, whereas in strong persons not merely do none of these things happen, but even a large quantity of bread or meat passes rapidly down.

And it is not only because the stomach is distended and loaded and because the fluid runs from one part of it to another accompanied by gurglings—it is not only for these reasons that one would judge that there was an unduly long continuance of the food in it, in those people who are so disposed, but also from the vomiting. Thus, there are some who vomit up every particle of what they have eaten, not after three or four hours, but actually in the middle of the night, a lengthy period having elapsed since their meal. Suppose you fill any animal whatsoever with liquid food—an experiment I have often carried out in pigs, to whom I give a sort of mess of wheaten flour and water, there after cutting them open after three or four hours; if you will do this yourself, you will find the food still in the stomach. For it is not chylification which determines the length of its stay here—since this can also be effected outside the stomach; the determining factor is digestion which is a different thing from chylification, as are blood-production and nutrition. For, just as it has been shown that these two processes depend upon a change of qualities, similarly also the digestion of food in the stomach involves a transmutation of it into the quality proper to that which is receiving nourishment. Then, when it is completely digested, the lower outlet opens and the food is quickly ejected through it, even if there should be amongst it abundance of stones, bones, grape-pips, or other things which cannot be reduced to chyle. And you may observe this yourself in an animal, if you will try to hit upon the time at which the descent of food from the stomach takes place.

But even if you should fail to discover the time, and nothing was yet passing down, and the food was still undergoing digestion in the stomach, still even then you would find dissection not without its uses.

You will observe, as we have just said, that the pylorus is accurately closed, and that the whole stomach is in a state of contraction upon the food very much as the womb contracts upon the foetus. For it is never possible to find a vacant space in the uterus, the stomach, or in either of the two bladders—that is, either in that called bile—receiving or in the other; whether their contents be abundant or scanty, their cavities are seen to be replete and full, owing to the fact that their coats contract constantly upon the contents—so long, at least, as the animal is in a natural condition. Now Erasistratus for some reason declares that it is the contractions of the stomach which are the cause of everything—that is to say, of the softening of the food, the removal of waste matter, and the absorption of the food when chylified [emulsified]. Now I have personally, on countless occasions, divided the peritoneum of a still living animal and have always found all the intestines contracting peristaltically upon their contents. The condition of the stomach, however, is found less simple; as regards the substances freshly swallowed, it had grasped these accurately both above and below, in fact at every point, and was as devoid of movement as though it had grown round and become united with the food. At the same time I found the pylorus persistently closed and accurately shut, like the os uteri on the foetus. In the cases, however, where digestion had been completed the pylorus had opened, and the stomach was undergoing peristaltic movements, similar to those of the intestines.

5 Thus all these facts agree that the stomach, uterus, and bladders possess certain inborn faculties which are retentive of their own proper qualities and eliminative of those that are foreign. For it has been already shown that the bladder by the liver draws bile into itself, while it is also quite obvious that it eliminates this daily into the stomach. Now, of course, if the eliminative were to succeed the attractive faculty and there were not a retentive faculty between the two, there would be found, on every occasion that animals were dissected, an equal quantity of bile in the gall-bladder. This, however, we do not find. For the bladder is sometimes observed to be very full, sometimes quite empty, while at other times you find in it various intermediate degrees of fulness, just as is the case with the other bladder—that which receives the urine; for even without resorting to anatomy we may observe that the urinary bladder continues to collect urine up to the time that it becomes uncomfortable through the increasing quantity of urine or the irritation caused by its acidity—the presumption thus being that there, too, there is a retentive faculty. Similarly, too, the stomach, when, as often happens, it is irritated by acidity, gets rid of the food, although still undigested, earlier than proper; or again, when oppressed by the quantity of its contents, or disordered from the co-existence of both conditions, it is seized with diarrhoea. Vomiting also is an affection of the upper [part of the] stomach analogous to diarrhoea, and it occurs when the stomach is overloaded or is unable to stand the quality of the food or surplus substances which it contains. Thus, when such a condition develops in the lower parts of the stomach, while the parts about the inlet are normal, it ends in diarrhoea, whereas if the condition is in the upper stomach, the lower parts being normal, it ends in vomiting.

6 This may often be seen clearly in those who are disinclined for food; when obliged to eat, they have not the strength to swallow, and, even if they force themselves to do so, they cannot retain the food, but at once vomit it up. And those especially who have a dislike to some particular kind of food, sometimes take it under compulsion, and then promptly bring it up; or, if they force themselves to keep it down, they are nauseated and feel their stomach turned up, and endeavouring to relieve itself of its discomfort. Thus, as was said at the beginning, all the observed facts testify that there must exist in almost all parts of the animal a certain inclination towards, or, so to speak, an appetite for their own special quality, and an aversion to, or, as it were, a hatred of the foreign quality. And it is natural that when they feel an inclination they should attract, and that when they feel aversion they should expel. From these facts, then, again, both the attractive and the propulsive faculties have been demonstrated to exist in everything. But if there be an inclination or attraction, there will also be some benefit derived; for no existing thing attracts anything else for the mere sake of attracting, but in order to benefit by what is acquired by the attraction. And of course it cannot benefit by it if it cannot retain it. Herein, then, again, the retentive faculty is shown to have its necessary origin: for the stomach obviously inclines towards its own proper qualities and turns away from those that are foreign to it. But if it aims at and attracts its food and benefits by it while retaining and contracting upon it, we may also expect that there will be some termination to the benefit received, and that thereafter will come the time for the exercise of the eliminative faculty.

7 But if the stomach both retains and benefits by its food, then it employs it for the end, for which it [the stomach] naturally exists. And it exists to partake of that which is of a quality befitting and proper to it. Thus it attracts all the most useful parts of the food in a vaporous and finely divided condition, storing this up in its own coats, and applying it to them. And when it is sufficiently full it puts away from it, as one might something troublesome, the rest of the food, this having itself meanwhile obtained some profit from its association with the stomach. For it is impossible for two bodies which are adapted for acting and being acted upon to come together without either both acting or being acted upon, or else one acting and the other being acted upon. For if their forces are equal they will act and be acted upon equally, and if the one be much superior in strength, it will exert its activity upon its passive neighbour; thus, while producing a great and appreciable effect, it will itself be acted upon either little or not at all. But it is herein also that the main difference lies between nourishing food and a deleterious drug; the latter masters the forces of the body, whereas the former is mastered by them. There cannot, then, be food which is suited for the animal which is not also correspondingly subdued by the qualities existing in the animal. And to be subdued means to undergo alteration.

Now, some parts are stronger in power and others weaker; therefore, while all will subdue the nutriment which is proper to the animal, they will not all do so equally. Thus the stomach will subdue and alter its food, but not to the same extent as will the liver, veins, arteries, and heart. We must therefore observe to what extent it does alter it. The alteration is more than that which occurs in the mouth, but less than that in the liver and veins. For the latter alteration changes the nutriment into the substance of blood, whereas that in the mouth obviously changes it into a new form, but certainly does not completely transmute it. This you may discover in the food which is left in the intervals between the teeth, and which remains there all night; the bread is not exactly bread, nor the meat meat, for they have a smell similar to that of the animal's mouth, and have been disintegrated and dissolved, and have had the qualities of the animal's flesh impressed upon them. And you may observe the extent of the alteration which occurs to food in the mouth if you will chew some corn and then apply it to an unripe [undigested] boil: you will see it rapidly transmuting—in fact entirely digesting—the boil, though it cannot do anything of the king if you mix it with water. And do not let this surprise you; this phlegm [saliva] in the mouth is also a cure for lichens [apparently skin-diseases in which a superficial crust (resembling the lichen on a tree-trunk) forms—e.g. psoriasis]; it even rapidly destroys scorpions; while, as regards the animals which emit venom, some it kills at once, and others after an interval; to all of them in any case it does great damage.

Now, the masticated food is all, firstly, soaked in and mixed up with this phlegm; and secondly, it is brought into contact with the actual skin of the mouth; thus it undergoes more change than the food which is wedged into the vacant space between the teeth. But just as masticated food is more altered than the latter kind, so is food which has been swallowed more altered than that which has been merely masticated. Indeed, there is no comparison between these two processes; we have only to consider what the stomach contains—phlegm, bile, pneuma, [innate] heat, and, indeed the whole substance of the stomach. And if one considers along with this the adjacent viscera like a lot of burning hearths around a great cauldron—to the right the liver, to the left the spleen, the heart above, and along with it the diaphragm (suspended and in a state of constant movement), and the omentum sheltering them all—you may believe what an extraordinary alteration it is which occurs in the food taken into the stomach. How could it easily become blood if it were not previously prepared by means of a change of this kind? It has already been shown that nothing is altered all at once from one quality to its opposite. How then could bread, beef, beans, or any other food turn into blood if they had not previously undergone some other alteration? And how could the faeces be generated right away in the small intestine? For what is there in this organ more potent in producing alteration than the factors in the stomach? Is it the number of the coats, or the way it is surrounded by neighbouring viscera, or the time that the food remains in it, or some kind of innate heat which it contains?

Most assuredly the intestines have the advantage of the stomach in none of these respects. For what possible reason, then, will objectors have it that bread may often remain a whole night in the stomach and still preserve its original qualities, whereas when once it is projected into the intestines, it straightway becomes ordure? For, if such a long period of time is incapable of altering it, neither will the short period be sufficient, or, if the latter is enough, surely the longer time will be much more so! Well, then, can it be that, while the nutriment does undergo an alteration in the stomach, this is a different kind of alteration and one which is not dependent on the nature of the organ which alters it? Or if it be an alteration of this latter kind, yet one perhaps which is not proper to the body of the animal? This is still more impossible. Digestion was shown to be nothing else than an alteration to the quality proper to that which is receiving nourishment. Since, then, this is what digestion means and since the nutriment has been shown to take on in the stomach a quality appropriate to the animal which is about to be nourished by it, it has been demonstrated adequately that nutriment does undergo digestion in the stomach. And Asclepiades is absurd when he states that the quality of the digested food never shows itself either in eructations or in the vomited matter, or on dissection. For of course the mere fact that the food smells of the body shows that it has undergone gastric digestion. But this man is so foolish that, when he hears the Ancients saying that the food is converted in the stomach into something "good," he thinks it proper to look out not for what is good in its possible effects, but for what is good to the taste: this is like saying that apples (for so one has to argue with him) become more apple-like [in flavour] in the stomach, or honey more honey-like! Erasistratus, however, is still more foolish and absurd, either through not perceiving in what sense the Ancients said that digestion is similar to the process of boiling, or because he purposely confused himself with sophistries. It is, he says, inconceivable that digestion, involving as it does such trifling warmth, should be related to the boiling process. This is as if we were to suppose that it was necessary to put the fires of Etna under the stomach before it could manage to alter the food; or else that, while it was capable of altering the food, it did not do this by virtue of its innate heat, which of course was moist, so that the word boil was used instead of bake.

What he ought to have done, if it was facts that he wished to dispute about, was to have tried to show, first and foremost, that the food is not transmuted or altered in quality by the stomach at all, and secondly, if he could not be confident of this, he ought to have tried to show that this alteration was not of any advantage to the animal. If, again, he were unable even to make this misrepresentation, he ought to have attempted to confute the postulate concerning the active principles—to show, in fact, that the functions taking place in the various parts do not depend in which the Warm, Cold, Dry, and Moist are mixed, but on some other factor. And if he had not the audacity to misrepresent facts even so far as this, still he should have tried at least to show that the Warm is not the most active of all the principles which play a part in things governed by Nature. But if he was unable to demonstrate this any more than any of the previous propositions, then he ought not to have made himself ridiculous by quarrelling uselessly with a mere name—as though Aristotle had not clearly stated in the fourth book of his *Meteorology,* as well as in many other passages, in what way digestion can be said to be allied to boiling, and also that the latter expression is not used in its primitive or strict sense. But, as has been frequently said already, the one starting-point of all this is a thorough-going enquiry into the question of the Warm, Cold, Dry and Moist; this Aristotle carried out in the second of his books *On Genesis and Destruction,* where he shows that all the transmutations and alterations throughout the body take place as a result of these principles. Erasistratus, however, advanced nothing against these or anything else that has been said above, but occupied himself merely with the word "boiling."

8 Thus, as regards digestion, even though he neglected everything else, he did at least attempt to prove his point—namely, that digestion in animals differs from boiling carried on outside; in regard to the question of deglutition, however, he did not go even so far as this. What are his words? *The stomach does not appear to exercise any traction.* Now the fact is that the stomach possesses two coats, which certainly exist for some purpose; they extend as far as the mouth, the internal one remaining throughout similar to what it is in the stomach, and the other one tending to become of a more fleshy nature in the gullet. Now simple observation will testify that these coats [the mucous and the muscular coats] have their fibres inserted in contrary directions. And, although Erasistratus did not attempt to say for what reason they are like this, I am going to do so. The inner coat has its fibres straight, since it exists for the purpose of traction. The outer coat has its fibres transverse, for the purpose of peristalsis. In fact, the movements of each of the mobile organs of the body depend on the setting of the fibres.

Now please test this assertion first in the muscles themselves; in these the fibres are most distinct, and their movements visible owing to their vigour. And after the muscles, pass to the physical organs, and you will see that they all move in correspondence with their fibres. This is why the fibres throughout the intestines are circular in both coats—they only contract peristaltically, they do not exercise traction. The stomach, again, has some of its fibres longitudinal for the purpose of traction and the others transverse for the purpose of peristalsis. For just as the movements in the muscles take place when each of the fibres becomes tightened and drawn towards its origin, such also is what happens in the stomach; when the transverse fibres tighten, the breadth of the cavity contained by them becomes less; and when the longitudinal fibres contract and draw in upon themselves, the length must necessarily be curtailed. This curtailment of length, indeed, is well seen in the act of swallowing: the larynx is seen to rise upwards to exactly the same degree that the gullet is drawn downwards; while, after the process of swallowing has been completed and the gullet is released from tension, the larynx can be clearly seen to again. This is because the inner coat of the stomach, which has the longitudinal fibres and which also lines the gullet and mouth, extends to the interior of the larynx, and it is thus impossible for it to be drawn down by the stomach without the larynx being involved in the traction.

Further, it will be found in Erasistratus's own writings that the circular fibres (by which the stomach as well as other parts performs its contractions) do not curtail its length, but contract and lessen its breadth. For he says that the stomach contracts peristaltically round the food during the whole period of digestion. But if it contracts, without in any way being diminished in length, this is because downward traction of the gullet is not a property of the movement of circular peristalsis. For what alone happens, as Erasistratus himself said, is that when the upper parts contract the lower ones dilate. And everyone knows that this can be plainly seen happening even in a dead man, if water be poured down his throat; this symptom results from the passage of matter through a narrow channel; it would be extraordinary if the channel did not dilate when a mass was passing through it. Obviously then the dilatation of the lower parts along with the contraction of the upper is common both to dead bodies, when anything whatsoever is passing through them, and to living ones, whether they contract peristaltically round their contents or attract them. Curtailment of length, on the other hand, is peculiar to organs which possess longitudinal fibres for the purpose of attraction. But the gullet was shown to be pulled down; for otherwise it would not have drawn upon the larynx.

It is therefore clear that the stomach attracts food by the gullet. Further, in vomiting, the mere passive conveyance of rejected matter up to the mouth will certainly itself suffice to keep open those parts of the oesophagus which are distended by the returned food; as it occupies each part in front [above], it first dilates this, and of course leaves the part behind [below] contracted. Thus, in this respect at least, the condition of the gullet is precisely similar to what it is in the act of swallowing. But there being no traction, the whole length remains equal in such cases. And for this reason it is easier to swallow than to vomit, for deglutition results the coats of the stomach being brought into action, the inner one exerting a pull and the outer one helping by peristalsis and propulsion, whereas emesis occurs from the outer coat alone functioning, without there being any kind of pull towards the mouth. For, although the swallowing of food is ordinarily preceded by a feeling of desire on the part from the mouth-parts for the experience; the two are opposite dispositions of the stomach itself; it yearns after and tends towards what is advantageous and proper to it, it loathes and rids itself of what is foreign. Thus the actual process of swallowing occurs very quickly in those who have a good appetite for such foods as are proper to the stomach; this organ obviously draws them in and down before they are masticated; whereas in the case of those who are forced to take a medicinal draught or who take food as medicine, the swallowing of these articles is accomplished with distress and difficulty.

From what has been said, then, it is clear that the inner coat of the stomach (that containing longitudinal fibres) exists for the purpose of exerting a pull to stomach, and that it is only in deglutition that it is active, whereas the external coat, which contains transverse fibres, has been so constituted in order that it may contract upon its contents and propel them forward; this coat furthermore, functions in vomiting no less than in swallowing. The truth of my statement is also borne out by what happens in the channae and synodonts; the stomachs of these animals are sometimes found in their mouths, as also Aristotle writes in his *History of Animals;* he also adds the cause of this: he says that it is owing to their voracity. The facts are as follows. In all animals, when the appetite is very intense, the stomach rises up, so that some people who have a clear perception of this condition say that their stomach "creeps out" of them; in others, who are still masticating their food and have not yet worked it up properly in the mouth, the stomach obviously snatches away the food from them against their will. In those animals, therefore, which are naturally voracious, in whom the mouth cavity is of generous proportions, and the stomach situated close to it (as in the case of the synodont and channae), it is in no way surprising that, when they are sufficiently hungry and are pursuing one of the smaller animals, and are just on the point of catching it, the stomach should, under the impulse of desire, spring into the mouth. And this cannot possibly take place in any other way than by the stomach drawing the food to itself by means of the gullet, as though by a hand. In fact, just as we ourselves, in our eagerness to grasp more quickly something lying before us, sometimes stretch out our whole bodies along with our hands, so also the stomach stretches itself forward along with the gullet, which is, as it were, its hand. And thus, in these animals in whom those three factors co-exist—an excessive propensity for food, a small gullet, and ample mouth proportions—in these, any slight tendency to movement forwards brings the whole stomach into the mouth. Now the constitution of the organs might itself suffice to give a naturalist an indication of their functions.

For Nature would never have purposelessly constructed the oesophagus of two coats with contrary dispositions; they must also have each been meant to have a different action. The Erasistratean school, however, are capable of anything rather than of recognizing the effects of Nature. Come, therefore, let us demonstrate to them by animal dissection as well that each of the two coats does exercise the activity which I have stated. Take an animal, then; lay bare the structures surrounding the gullet, without severing any of the nerves, arteries, or veins which are there situated; next divide with vertical incisions, from the lower jaw to the thorax, the outer coat of the oesophagus (that containing transverse fibres); then give the animal food and you will see that it still swallows although the peristaltic function has been abolished. If, again, in another animal, you cut through both coats with transverse incisions, you will observe that this animal swallows although the inner coat is no longer functioning.

From this it is clear that the animal can also swallow by either of the two coats, although not so well as by both. For the following also, in addition to other points, may be distinctly observed in the dissection which I have described—that during deglutition the gullet becomes slightly filled with air which is swallowed along with the food, and that, when the outer coat is contracting, this air is easily forced with the food into the stomach, but that, when there only exists an inner coat, the air impedes the conveyance of food, by distending this coat and hindering its action. But Erasistratus said nothing about this, nor did he point out that the oblique situation of the gullet clearly confutes the teaching of those who hold that it is simply by virtue of the impulse from above that food which is swallowed reaches the stomach. The only correct thing he said was that many of the longnecked animals bend down to swallow. Hence, clearly, the observed fact does not show how we swallow is not due merely to the impulse from above; it is yet, however, not clear whether it results from the food being attracted by the stomach, or conducted by the gullet. For our part, however, having enumerated all the different considerations—those based on the constitution of the organs, as well as those based on the other symptoms which, as just mentioned, occur both before and after the gullet has been exposed—we have thus sufficiently proved that the inner coat exists for the purpose of attraction and the outer for the purpose of propulsion. Now the original task we set before ourselves was to demonstrate that the retentive faculty exists in every one of the organs, just as in the previous book we proved the existence of the attractive, and, over and above this, the alterative faculty. Thus, in the natural course of our argument, we have demonstrated these four faculties existing in the stomach—the attractive faculty in connection with swallowing, the retentive with digestion, the expulsive with vomiting and with the descent of digested food into the small intestine—and digestion itself we have shown to be a process of alteration.

9 Concerning the spleen, also, we shall therefore have no further doubts as to whether it attracts what is proper to it, rejects what is foreign, and has a natural power of altering and retaining all that it attracts; nor shall we be in any doubt as to the liver, veins, arteries, heart, or any other organ. For these four faculties have been shown to be necessary for every part which is to be nourished; this is why we have called these faculties the handmaids of nutrition. For just as human faeces are most pleasing to dogs, so the residual matters from the liver are, some of them, proper to the spleen, others to the gall-bladder, and others to the kidneys.

10 I should not have cared to say anything further as to the origin of these [surplus substances] after Hippocrates, Plato, Aristotle, Diocles, Praxagoras, and Philotimus, nor indeed should I even have said anything about the faculties, if any of our predecessors had worked out this subject thoroughly. While, however, the statements which the Ancients made on these points were correct, they yet omitted to defend their statements with logical proofs; of course they never suspected that there could be sophists so shameless as to try to contradict obvious facts. More recent physicians, again, have been partly conquered by the sophistries of these fellows and have given credence to them; whilst others who attempted to argue with them appear to me to lack to a great extent the power of the Ancients. For this reason I have attempted to put together my arguments in the way in which it seems to me the Ancients, had any of them been still alive, would have done, in opposition to those who would overturn the finest doctrines of our art. I am not, however, unaware that I shall achieve either nothing at all or else very little. For I find that a great many things which have been conclusively demonstrated by the Ancients are unintelligible to the bulk of the Moderns owing to their ignorance—nay, that, by reason of their laziness, they will not even make an attempt to comprehend them; and even in any of them have understood them, they have not given them impartial examination. The fact is that he whose purpose is to know anything better than the multitude do must far surpass all others both as regards his nature and his early training. And when he reaches early adolescence he must become possessed with an ardent love for truth, like one inspired; neither day nor night may he cease to urge and strain himself in order to learn thoroughly all that has been said by the most illustrious of the Ancients. And when he has learnt this, then for a prolonged period he must test and prove it, observing what part of it is in agreement, and what in disagreement with obvious fact; thus he will choose this and turn away from that. To such an one my hope has been that my treatise would prove of the very greatest assistance. . . . Still, such people may be expected to be quite few in number, while, as for the others, this book will be as superfluous to them as a tale told to an ass.

11 For the sake, then, of those who are aiming at truth, we must complete this treatise by adding what is still wanting in it. Now, in people who are very hungry, the stomach obviously attracts or draws down the food before it has been thoroughly softened in the mouth, whilst in those who have no appetite or who are being forced to eat, the stomach is displeased and rejects the food. And in a similar way of the other organs possesses both faculties—that of attracting what is proper to it, and that of rejecting what is foreign. Thus, even if there be any organ which consists of only one coat (such as the two bladders, the uterus, and the veins), it yet possesses both kinds of fibres, the longitudinal and the transverse. But further, there are fibres of a third kind—the oblique—which are much fewer in number than the two kinds already spoken of. In the organs consisting of two coats this kind of fibre is found in the one coat only, mixed with the longitudinal fibres; but in the organs composed of one coat it is found along with the other two kinds. Now, these are of the greatest help to the action of the faculty which we have named retentive. For during this period the part needs to be tightly contracted and stretched over its contents at every point—the stomach during the whole period of digestion, and the uterus during that of gestation. Thus too, the coat of a vein, being single, consists of various kinds of fibres; whilst the outer coat of an artery consists of circular fibres, and its inner coat mostly of longitudinal fibres, but with a few oblique ones also amongst them. Veins thus resemble the uterus or the bladder as regards the arrangement of their fibres, even though they are deficient in thickness; similarly arteries resemble the stomach. Alone of all organs the intestines consist of two coats of which both have their fibres transverse. Now the proof that it was for the best that all the organs should be naturally such as they are (that, for instance, the intestines should be composed of two coats) belongs to the subject of the use of parts; thus we must not now desire to hear about matters of this kind nor why the anatomists are at variance regarding the number of coats in each organ. For these questions have been sufficiently discussed in the treatise *On Disagreement in Anatomy*. And the problem as to why each organ has such and such a character will be discussed in the treatise *On the Use of Parts.*

12 It is not, however, our business to discuss either of these questions here, but to consider duly the natural faculties, which, to the number of four, exist in each organ. Returning then, to this point, let us recall what has already been said, and set a crown to the whole subject by adding what is still wanting. For when every part of the animal has been shewn to draw into itself the juice which is proper to it (this being practically the first of the natural faculties), the next point to realize is that the part does not get rid either of this attracted nutriment as a whole, or even of any superfluous portion of it, until either the organ itself, or the major part of its contents also have their condition reversed. Thus, when the stomach is sufficiently filled with the food and has absorbed and stored away the most useful part of it in its own coats, it then rejects the rest like an alien burden. The same happens to bladders, when the matter attracted into them begins to give trouble either because it distends them through its quantity or irritates them by its quality. And this also happens in the case of the uterus; for it is either because it can no longer bear to be stretched that it strives to relieve itself of it annoyance, or else because it is irritated by the quality of the fluids poured into it.

Now both of these conditions sometimes occur with actual violence, and then miscarriage takes place. But for the most part they happen in a normal way, this being then called not miscarriage but delivery or parturition. Now abortifacient drugs or certain other conditions which destroy the embryo or rupture certain of its membranes are followed by abortion, and similarly also when the uterus is in pain from being in a bad state of tension; and, as has been well said by Hippocrates, excessive movement on the part of the embryo itself brings on labor. Now pain is common to all these conditions, and of this there are three possible causes—either excessive bulk, or weight, or irritation; bulk when the uterus can no longer support the stretching, weight when the contents surpass its strength, and irritation when the fluids which had previously been pent up in the membranes, flow out, on the rupture of these, into the uterus itself, or else when the whole foetus perishes, putrefies, and is resolved into pernicious ichors, and so irritates and bites the coat of the uterus. In all organs, then, both their natural effects and their disorders and maladies plainly take place on analogous lines, some so clearly and manifestly as to need no demonstration, and others less plainly, although not entirely unrecognizable to those who are willing to pay attention.

Thus, to take the case of the stomach: the irritation is evident here because this organ possesses most sensibility, and among its other affections those producing nausea and the so-called heartburn clearly demonstrate the eliminative faculty which expels foreign matter. So also in the case of the uterus and the urinary bladder; this latter also may be plainly observed to receive and accumulate fluid until it is so stretched by the amount of this as to be incapable of enduring the pain; or it may be the quality of the urine which irritates it; for every superfluous substance which lingers in the body must obviously putrefy, some in a shorter, and some in a longer time, and thus it becomes pungent, acrid, and burdensome to the organ which contains it. This does not apply, however, in the case of the bladder alongside the liver, whence it is clear that it possesses fewer nerves than do the other organs.

Here too, however, at least the physiologist must discover an analogy. For since it was shown that the gall-bladder attracts its own special juice, so as to be often found full, and that it discharges it soon after, this desire to discharge must be either due to the fact that it is burdened by the quantity or that the bile has changed in quality to pungent and acrid. For while food does not change its original quality so fast that it is already ordure as soon as it falls into the small intestine, on the other hand the bile even more readily than the urine becomes altered in quality as soon as ever it leaves the veins, and rapidly undergoes change and putrefaction. Now, if there be clear evidence in relation to the uterus, stomach, and intestines, as well as to the urinary bladder, that there is either some distention, irritation, or burden inciting each of these organs to elimination, there is no difficulty in imagining this in the case of the gall-bladder also, as well as in the other organs,—to which obviously the arteries and veins also belong.

13 Nor is there any further difficulty in ascertaining that it is through the same channel that both attraction and discharge take place at different times. For obviously the inlet to the stomach does not merely conduct food and drink into this organ, but in the condition of nausea it performs the neck of the bladder which is beside the liver, albeit single, both fills and empties the bladder. Similarly the canal of the uterus affords an entrance to the semen and an exit to the foetus. But in this latter case, again, whilst the eliminative faculty is evident, the attractive faculty is not so obvious to most people. It is, however, the cervix which Hippocrates blames for inertia of the uterus when he says: *Its orifice has no power of attracting semen.* Erasistratus, however, and Asclepiades reached such heights of wisdom that they deprived not merely the stomach and the womb of this faculty but also the bladder by the liver, and the kidneys as well. I have, however, pointed out in the first book that it is impossible to assign any other cause for the secretion of urine or bile. Now, when we find that the uterus, the stomach and the bladder by the liver carry out attraction and expulsion through one and the same duct, we need no longer feel surprised that Nature should also frequently discharge waste-substances into the stomach through the veins. Still less need we be astonished if a certain amount of the food should, during long fasts, be drawn back from the liver into the stomach through the same veins by which it was yielded up to the liver during absorption of nutriment. To disbelieve such things would of course be like refusing to believe that purgative drugs draw their appropriate humors from all over the body by the same stomata through which absorption previously takes place, and to look for separate stomata for absorption and purgation respectively.

As a matter of fact one and the same stomata subserves two distinct faculties, and these exercise their pull at different times in opposite directions—first it subserves the pull of the liver and, during catharsis, that of the drug. What is there surprising, then, in the fact that the veins situated between the liver and the region of the stomach fulfil a double service or purpose? Thus, when there is abundance of nutriment contained in the food-canal, it is carried up to the liver by the veins mentioned; and when the canal is empty and in need of nutriment, this is again attracted from the liver by the same veins. For everything appears to attract from and to go shares with everything else, and, as the most divine Hippocrates has said, there would seem to be a consensus in the movements of fluids and vapours. Thus the stronger draws and the weaker is evacuated. Now, one part is weaker or stronger than another either absolutely, by nature, and in all cases, or else it becomes so in such and such a particular instance. Thus, by nature and in all men alike, the heart is stronger than the liver at attracting what is serviceable to it and rejecting what is not so; similarly the liver is stronger than the intestines and stomach, and the arteries than the veins. In each of us personally, however, liver has stronger drawing power at one time, and the stomach at another. For when there is much nutriment contained in the alimentary canal and the appetite and craving of the liver is violent, then the viscus exerts far the strongest traction. Again, when the liver is full and distended and the stomach empty and in need, then the force of the traction shifts to the latter. Suppose we had some food in our hands and were snatching it from one another; if we were equally in want, the stronger would be likely to prevail, but if he had satisfied his appetite, and was holding what was over carelessly, or was anxious to share it with somebody, and if the weaker was excessively desirous of it, there would be nothing to prevent the latter from getting it all. In a similar manner the stomach easily attracts nutriment from the liver when it [the stomach] has a sufficiently strong craving for it, and the appetite of the viscus is satisfied. And sometimes the surplusage of nutriment in the liver is a reason why the animal is not hungry; for when the stomach has better and more available food it requires nothing from extraneous sources, but if ever it is in need and is at a loss how to supply the need, it becomes filled with waste-matters; these are certain biliary, phlegmatic [mucous] and serous fluids, and are the only substances that the liver yields in response to the traction of the stomach, on the occasions when the latter too is in want of nutriment.

Now, just as the parts draw food from each other, so also they sometimes deposit their excess substances in each other, and just as the stronger prevailed when the two were exercising traction, so it is also when they are depositing; this is the cause of the so-called fluxions, for every part has a definite inborn tension, by virtue of which it expels its superfluities, and, therefore, when one of these parts,—owing, of course, to some special condition—becomes weaker, there will necessarily be a confluence into it of the superfluities from all the other parts. The strongest part deposits its surplus matter in all the parts near it; these again in other parts which are weaker; these next into yet others; and this goes on for a long time, until the superfluity, being driven from one part into another, comes to rest in one of the weakest of it all; it cannot flow from this into another part, because none of the stronger ones will receive it, while the affected part is unable to drive it away. When, however, we come to deal again with the origin and cure of disease, it will be possible to find there also abundant proofs of all that we have correctly indicated in this book. For the present, however, let us resume again the task that lay before us, i.e. to show that there is nothing surprising in nutriment coming from the liver to the intestines and stomach by way of the very veins through which it had previously been yielded up from these organs into the liver. And in many people who have suddenly and completely given up active exercise, or who have had a limb cut off, there occurs at certain periods an evacuation of blood by way of the intestines—as Hippocrates has also pointed out somewhere. This causes no further trouble but sharply purges the whole body and evacuates the plethoras; the passage of the superfluities is effected, of course, through the same veins by which absorption took place.

Frequently also in disease Nature purges the animal through these same veins—although in this case the discharge is not sanguineous, but corresponds to the humour which is at fault. Thus in cholera the entire body is evacuated by way of the veins leading to the intestines and stomach. To imagine that matter of different kinds is carried in one direction only would characterise a man who was entirely ignorant of all the natural faculties, and particularly of the eliminative faculty, which is the opposite of the attractive. For opposite movements of matter, active and passive, must necessarily follow opposite faculties; that is to say, every part, after it has attracted its special nutrient juice and has retained and taken benefit of it hastens to get rid of all the surplusage as quickly and effectively as possible, and this it does in accordance with the mechanical tendency of this surplus matter. Hence the stomach clears away by vomiting those superfluities which come to the surface of its contents, whilst the sediment it clears away by diarrhoea. And when the animal becomes sick, this means that the stomach is striving to be evacuated by vomiting. And the expulsive faculty has in it so violent and forcible an element that in case of ileus [volvulus], when the lower exist is completely closed, vomiting of faeces occurs; yet such surplus matter could not be emitted from the mouth without having first traversed the whole of the small intestine, the jejunum, the pylorus, the stomach, and the oesophagus. What is there to wonder at, then, if something should also be transferred from the extreme skin-surface and so reach the intestines and stomach? This also was pointed out to us by Hippocrates, who maintained that not merely pneuma or excess-matter, but actual nutriment is brought down from the outer surface to the original place from which it was taken up.

For the slightest mechanical movements determine this expulsive faculty, which apparently acts through the transverse fibres, and which is very rapidly transmitted from the source of motion to the opposite extremities. It is, therefore, neither unlikely nor impossible that, when the part adjoining the skin becomes suddenly oppressed by an unwonted cold, it should at once be weakened and should find that the liquid previously deposited beside it without discomfort had now become more of a burden than a source of nutrition, and should therefore strive to put it away. Finally, seeing that the passage outwards was shut off by the condensation [of tissue], it would turn to the remaining exit and would thus forcibly expel all the waste-matter at once into the adjacent part; this would do the same to the part following it; and the process would not cease until the transference finally terminated at the inner of the veins. Now, movements like these come to an end fairly soon, but those resulting from internal irritants (e.g., in the administration of purgative drugs or in cholera) become much stronger and more lasting; they persist as long as the condition of things about the mouths of the veins continues, that is, so long as these continue to attract what is adjacent. For this condition causes evacuation of the contiguous part, and that again of the part next to it, and this never stops until the extreme surface is reached; thus, as each part keeps passing on matter to its neighbour, the original affection very quickly arrives at the extreme termination. Now this is also the case in ileus; the inflamed intestine is unable to support either the weight or the acridity of the waste substances and so does its best to excrete them, in fact to drive them as far away as possible. And, being prevented from effecting an expulsion downwards when the severest part of the inflammation is there, it expels the matter into the adjoining part of the intestines situated above. Thus the tendency of the eliminative faculty is step by step upwards, until the superfluities reach the mouth. Now this will be also spoken of at greater length in my treatise on disease.

For the present, however, I think I have shown clearly that there is a universal conveyance or transference from one thing to another, and that, as Hippocrates used to say, there exists in everything a consensus in the movement of air and fluids. And I do not think that anyone, however slow his intellect, will now be at a loss to understand any of these points,—how, for instance, the stomach or intestines get nourished, or in what manner anything makes its way inwards from the outer surface of the body. Seeing that all parts have the faculty of attracting what is suitable or well-disposed and of eliminating what is troublesome or irritating, it is not surprising that opposite movements should occur in them consecutively—as may be clearly seen in the case of the heart, in the various arteries, in the thorax, and lungs. In all these the active movements of the organs and therewith the passive movements of [their contained] matters may be seen taking place almost every second in opposite directions.

Now, you are not astonished when the trachea-artery alternately draws air into the lungs and gives it out, and when the nostrils and the whole mouth act similarly; nor do you think it strange or paradoxical that the air is dismissed through the very channel by which it was admitted just before. Do you, then, feel a difficulty in the case of the veins which pass down from the liver into the stomach and intestines, and do you think it strange that nutriment should at once be yielded up to the liver and drawn back from it into the stomach by the same veins? You must define what you mean by this expression "at once." If you mean "at the same time" this is not what we ourselves say; for just as we take in a breath at one moment and give it out again at another, so at one time the liver draws nutriment from the stomach, and at another the stomach from the liver. But if your expression "at once" means that in one and the same animal a single organ subserves the transport of matter in opposite directions, and if it is this which disturbs you, consider inspiration and expiration. For of course these also take place through the same organs, albeit they differ in their manner of movement, and in the way in which the matter is conveyed through them. Now the lungs, the thorax, the arteries rough and smooth, the heart, the mouth, and the nostrils reverse their movements at very short intervals and change the direction of the matters they contain.

On the other hand, the veins which pass down from the liver to the intestines and stomach reverse the direction not at such short intervals, but sometimes once in many days. The whole matter, in fact, is as follows: Each of the organs draws to itself the nutriment alongside it, and devours all the useful fluid in it, until it is thoroughly satisfied; this nutriment, as I have already shown, it stores up in itself, afterwards making it adhere and then assimilating it—that is, it becomes nourished by it. For it has been demonstrated with sufficient clearness already that there is something which necessarily precedes actual nutrition, namely adhesion, and that before this again comes presentation. Thus as in the case of the animals themselves the end of eating is that the stomach should be filled, similarly in the case of each of the parts, the end of presentation is the filling of this part with its appropriate liquid. Since, therefore, every part has, like the stomach, a craving to be nourished, it too envelops its nutriment and clasps it all round as the stomach does. And this [action of the stomach], as has been already said, is necessarily followed by the digestion of the food, although it is not to make it suitable for the other parts that the stomach contracts upon it; if it did so, it would no longer be a physiological organ, but an animal possessing reason and intelligence, with the power of choosing the better [of two alternatives].

But while the stomach contracts for the reason that the whole body possesses a power of attracting and of utilising appropriate qualities, as has already been explained, it also happens that, in this process, the food undergoes alteration; further, when filled and saturated with the fluid pabulum from the food, it thereafter looks on the food as a burden; thus it at once gets of the excess—that is to say, drives it gets downwards—itself turning to another task, namely that of causing adhesion. And during this time, while the nutriment is passing along the whole length of the intestine, it is caught up by the vessels which pass into the intestine; as we shall shortly demonstrate, most of it is seized by the veins, but a little also by the arteries; at this stage also it becomes presented to the coats of the intestines. Now imagine the whole economy of nutrition divided into three periods. Suppose that in the first period the nutriment remains in the stomach and is digested and presented to the stomach until satiety is reached, also that some of it is taken up from the stomach to the liver. During the second period it passes along the intestines and becomes presented both to them and to the liver—again until the stage of satiety—while a small part of it is carried all over the body. During this period, also imagine that what was presented to the stomach in the first period becomes now adherent to it. During the third period the stomach has reached the stage of receiving nourishment; it now entirely assimilates everything that had become adherent to it: at the same time in the intestines and liver there takes place adhesion of what had been before presented, while dispersal [anadosis] is taking place to all parts of the body, as also presentation.

Now, if the animal takes food immediately after these [three stages] then, during the time that the stomach is again digesting and getting the benefit of this by presenting all the useful part of it to its own coats, the intestines will be engaged in final assimilation of the juices which have adhered to them, and so also will the liver: while in the various parts of the body there will be taking place adhesion of the portions of nutriment presented. And if the stomach is forced to remain without food during this time, it will draw its nutriment from the veins in the mesentery and liver; for it will not do so from the actual body of the liver (by body of the liver I mean first and foremost its flesh proper, and after this all the vessels contained in it), for it is irrational to suppose that one part would draw away from another part the juice already contained in it, especially when adhesion and final assimilation of that juice were already taking place; the juice, however, that is in the cavity of the veins will be abstracted by the part which is stronger and more in need. It is in this way, therefore, that the stomach, when it is in need of nourishment and the animal has nothing to eat, seizes it from the veins in the liver. Also in the case of the spleen we have shown in a former passage how it draws all material from the liver that tends to be thick, and by working it up converts it into more useful matter. There is nothing surprising, therefore, if, in the present instance also, some of this should be drawn from the spleen into such organs as communicate with it by veins, e.g. the omentum, mesentery, small intestine, colon, and the stomach itself. Nor is it surprising that the spleen should disgorge its surplus matters into the stomach at one time, while at another time it should draw some of its appropriate nutriment from the stomach.

For, as has already been said, speaking generally, everything has the power at different times of attracting from and of adding to everything else. What happens is just as if you might imagine a number of animals helping themselves at will to a plentiful common stock of food; some will naturally be eating when others have stopped, some will be on the point of stopping when others are beginning, some eating together, and others in succession. Yes, by Zeus! and one will often be plundering another, if he be in need while the other has an abundant supply ready to hand. Thus it is in no way surprising that matter should make its way back from the outer surface of the body to the interior, or should be carried from the liver and spleen into the stomach by the same vessels by which it was carried in the reverse direction. In the case of the arteries this is clear enough, as also in the case of heart, thorax, and lungs; for, since all of these dilate and contract alternately, it must needs be that matter is subsequently discharged back into the parts from which it was previously drawn. Now Nature foresaw this necessity, and provided the cardiac openings of the vessels with membranous attachments, to prevent their contents from being carried backwards. How and in what manner this takes place will be stated in my work *On the Use of Parts,* where among other things I show that it is impossible for the openings of the vessels to be closed so accurately that nothing at all can run back. Thus it is inevitable that the reflux into the venous artery (as will also be made clear in the work mentioned) should be much greater than through the other openings. But what it is important for our present purpose to recognise is that every thing possessing a large and appreciable cavity must, when it dilates, abstract matter from all its neighbours, and, when it contracts, must squeeze matter back into them. This should all be clear from what has already been said in this treatise and from what Erasistratus and I myself have demonstrated elsewhere respecting the tendency of a vacuum to become refilled.

14 And further, it has been shown in other treatises that all the arteries possess a power which derives from the heart, and by virtue of which they dilate and contract. Put together, therefore, the two facts—that the arteries have this motion, and that everything, when it dilates, draws neighbouring matter into itself—and you will find nothing strange in the fact that those arteries which reach the skin draw in the outer air when they dilate, while those which anastomose at any point with the veins attract the thinnest and most vaporous part of the blood which these contain, and as for those arteries which are near the heart, it is on the heart itself that they exert their traction. For, by virtue of the tendency by which a vacuum becomes refilled, the lightest and thinnest part obeys the tendency before that which is heavier and thicker. Now the lightest and thinnest of anything in the body is firstly pneuma, secondly vapour, and in the third place that part of the blood which has been accurately elaborated and refined.

These, then, are what the arteries draw into themselves on every side; those arteries which reach the skin draw in the outer air (this being near them and one of the lightest of things); as to the other arteries, those which pass up from the heart into the neck, and that which lies along the spine, as also such arteries as are near these—draw mostly from the heart itself; and those which are farther from the heart and skin necessarily draw the lightest part of the blood out of the veins. So also the traction exercised by the diastole of the arteries which go to the stomach and intestines takes place at the expense of the heart itself and the numerous veins in its neighbourhood; for these arteries cannot get anything worth speaking of from the thick heavy nutriment contained in the intestines and stomach, since they first become filled with lighter elements. For if you let down a tube into a vessel full of water and sand, and suck the air out of the tube with your mouth, the sand cannot come up to you before the water, for in accordance with the principle of the refilling of a vacuum the lighter matter is always the first to succeed to the evacuation.

15 It is not to be wondered at, therefore, that only a very little [nutrient matter] such, namely, as has been accurately elaborated—gets from the stomach into the arteries, since these first become filled with lighter matter. We must understand that there are two kinds of attraction, that by which a vacuum becomes refilled and that caused by appropriateness of quality; air is drawn into bellows in one way, and iron by the lodestone in another. And we must also understand that the traction which results from evacuation acts primarily on what is light, whilst that from appropriateness of quality acts frequently, it may be, on what is heavier (if this should be naturally more nearly related). Therefore, in the case of the heart and the arteries, it is in so far as they are hollow organs, capable of diastole, that they always attract the lighter matter first, while, in so far as they require nourishment, it is actually into their coats (which are the real bodies of these organs) that the appropriate matter is drawn.

Of the blood, then, which is taken into their cavities when they dilate, that part which is most proper to them and most able to afford nourishment is attracted by their actual coats. Now, apart from what has been said, the following is sufficient proof that something is taken over from the veins into the arteries. If you will kill an animal by cutting through a number of its large arteries, you will find the veins becoming empty along with the arteries: now, this could never occur if there were not anastomoses between them. Similarly, also, in the heart iself, the thinnest portion of the blood is drawn from the right ventricle into the left, owing to there being perforations in the septum between them: these can be seen for a great part [of their length]; they are like a kind of fossae [pits] with wide mouths, and they get constantly narrower; it is not possible, however, actually to observe their extreme terminations, owing both to the smallness of these and to the fact that when the animal is dead all the parts are chilled and shrunken. Here, too, however, our argument, starting from the principle that nothing is done by Nature in vain, discovers these anastomoses between the ventricles of the heart; for it could not be at random and by chance that there occurred fossae ending thus in narrow terminations. And secondly [the presence of these anastomoses has been assumed] from the fact that, of the two orifices in the right ventricle, the one conducting blood in and the other out, the former is much the larger. For, the fact that the insertion of the vena cava into the heart is larger than the vein which is inserted into the lungs suggests that not all the blood which the vena cava gives to the heart is driven away again from the heart to the lungs.

Nor can it be said that any of the blood is expended in the nourishment of the actual body of the heart, since there is another vein which breaks up in it and which does not take its origin nor get its share of the blood from the heart itself. And even if a certain amount is so expended, still the vein leading to the lungs is not to such a slight extent smaller than that inserted into the heart as to make it likely that the blood is used as nutriment for the heart: the disparity is much too great for such an explanation. It is, therefore, clear that something is taken over into the left ventricle. Moreover, of the two vessels connected with it, that which brings pneuma from the lungs is much smaller than the great outgrowing artery from which the arteries all over the body originate; this would suggest that it not merely gets pneuma from the lungs, but that it also gets blood from the right ventricle through the anastomoses mentioned. Now it belongs to the treatise *On the Use of Parts* to show that it was best that some parts of the body should be nourished by pure, thin, and vaporous blood, and others by thick, turbid blood, and that in this matter also Nature has overlooked nothing. Thus it is not desirable that these matters should be further discussed. Having mentioned, however, that there are two kinds of attraction, certain bodies exerting attraction along wide channels during diastole (by virtue of the principle by which a vacuum becomes refilled) and others exerting it by virtue of their appropriateness of quality, we must next remark that the former bodies can attract even from a distance, while the latter can only do so from among things which are quite close to them; the very longest tube let down into water can easily draw up the liquid to the mouth, but if you withdraw iron to a distance from the lodestone or corn from the jar (an instance of this kind has in fact been already given) no further attraction can take place. This you can observe most clearly in connection with garden conduits. For a certain amount of moisture is distributed from these into every part lying close at hand but it cannot reach those lying farther off: therefore one has to arrange the flow of water into all parts of the garden by cutting a number of small channels leading from the large one. The intervening spaces between these small channels are made of such a size as will, presumably, best allow them [the spaces] to satisfy their needs by drawing from the liquid which flows to them from every side.

So also is it in the bodies of animals. Numerous conduits distributed through the various limbs bring them pure blood, much like the garden water-supply, and, further, the intervals between these conduits have been wonderfully arranged by Nature from the outset so that the intervening parts should be plentifully provided for when absorbing blood, and that they should never be deluged by a quantity of superfluous fluid running in at unsuitable times. For the way in which they obtain nourishment is somewhat as follows. In the body which is continuous throughout, such as Erasistratus supposes his simple vessel to be, it is the superficial parts which are the first to make use of the nutriment with which they are brought into contact; then the parts coming next draw up their share from these by virtue of their contiguity; and again others from these; and this does not stop until the quality of the nutrient substance has been distributed among all parts of the corpuscle in question. And for such parts as need the humour which is destined to nourish them to be altered still further, Nature has provided a kind of storehouse, either in the form of a central cavity or else as separate caverns, or something analogous to caverns. Thus the flesh of the viscera and of the muscles is nourished from the blood directly, this having undergone merely a slight alteration; the bones, however, in order to be nourished, very great change, and what blood is to flesh marrow is to bone; in the case of the small bones, which do not possess central cavities, this marrow is distributed in their caverns, whereas in the larger bones which do contain central cavities the marrow is all concentrated in these. For as was pointed out in the first book, things having a similar substance can easily change into one another, whereas it is impossible for those which are very different to be assimilated to one another without intermediate stages.

Such a one in respect to cartilage is the myxoid substance which surrounds it, and in respect to ligaments, membranes, and nerves the viscous liquid dispersed inside them; for each of these consists of numerous fibres, which are homogeneous—in fact, actual sensible elements; and in the intervals between these fibres is dispersed the humous most suited for nutrition; this they draw from the blood in the veins, choosing the most appropriate possible, and now they are assimilating it step by step and changing it into their own substance. All these considerations, then, agree with one another, and bear sufficient witness to the truth of what has been already demonstrated; there is thus no need to prolong the discussion further. For, from what has been said, anyone can readily discover in what way all the particular [vital activites] come about. For instance, we could in this way ascertain why it is that in the case of many people who are partaking freely of wine, the fluid which they have drunk is rapidly absorbed throughout the body and almost the whole of it is passed by the kidneys within a very short time. For here, too, the rapidity with which the fluid is absorbed depends on appropriateness of quality, on the thinness of the fluid, on the width of the vessels and their mouths, and on the efficiency of the attractive faculty. The parts situated near the alimentary canal, by virtue of their appropriateness of quality, draw in the imbibed food for their own purposes, then the parts next to them in their turn snatch it away, then those next again take it from these, until it reaches the vena cava, whence finally the kidneys attract that part of it which is proper to them. Thus it is in no way surprising that wine is taken up more rapidly than water, owing to its appropriateness of quality, and, further, that the white clear kind of wine is absorbed more rapidly owing to its thinness, while black turbid wine is checked on the way and retarded because of its thickness. These facts, also, will afford abundant proof of what has already been said about the arteries; everywhere, in fact, such blood as is both specifically appropriate and at the same time thin in consistency answers more readily to their traction than does blood which is not so; this is why the arteries which, in their diastole, absorb vapour, pneuma, and thin blood attract either none at all or very little of the juices contained in the stomach and intestines.